Atlas of
Regional
Anesthesia

Atlas of
Regional
Anesthesia

Jordan Katz, M.D.
Professor, Department of Anesthesiology
University of California, San Diego
Staff Anesthesiologist
University Hospital and
Veterans Administration Medical Center
San Diego, California

**Illustrations by
John W. Brown, Cypress, California**

APPLETON & LANGE
Norwalk, Connecticut/San Mateo, California

Copyright © 1985 by Appleton-Century-Crofts
A Publishing Division of Prentice-Hall

91 / 10 9 8 7 6 5 4

Published simultaneously in Great Britain by Prentice-Hall International (UK) Limited, London; simultaneously in Australia by Prentice-Hall of Australia, Pty. Ltd., Sydney; simultaneously in Southeast Asia by Prentice-Hall of Southeast Asia (Pte.) Ltd., Singapore; and simultaneously in New Zealand by Whitehall Books Ltd., Wellington, New Zealand.

Distributed by:
Prentice-Hall Canada, Inc.
Prentice-Hall Hispanoamericana, S.A., Mexico
Prentice-Hall of India Private Limited, New Delhi
Prentice-Hall of Japan, Inc., Tokyo
Editora Prentice-Hall do Brasil Ltda., Rio de Janeiro

Library of Congress Cataloging in Publication Data

Katz, Jordan.
    Atlas of regional anesthesia.

    Includes index.
    1. Conduction anesthesia—Atlases.   I. Title.
RD85.C6K28   1985   617'.964   85-3953
ISBN 0-8385-0455-8

ISBN (US only): 0-8385-0455-8
ISBN (Outside the US): 0-8385-0127-3
Design: Jean M. Sabato-Morley

PRINTED IN THE UNITED STATES OF AMERICA

To Ruby
Cum Te Semper

Contents

Preface

The bases for nerve block analgesia have evolved over the last 100 years. In preparing this manuscript I was greatly impressed by the detailed information presented in several older texts, which, in reality, laid the groundwork for many of our current techniques. Several of these earlier endeavors stand out: Braun's *Die Lokal Anasthesie,* Labat's *Regional Anesthesia,* Pitkin's *Conduction Anesthesia,* Bonica's *Management of Pain,* and Moore's *Regional Block.* In addition, the recent text *Neural Blockade* by Cousins and Bridenbaugh is a significant contribution.

Contact with several individuals produced the additional stimulus necessary for me to write this atlas. Three in particular must be mentioned—Harold Carron, Alon Winnie, and Prithvi Raj.

Dr. Terry Davidson provided significant input for several of the head and neck blocks. The facilities at Linköping University, Department of Anesthesia were used extensively in the research for this book.

To John W. Brown a special debt of gratitude is necessary. His many long hours of work and dedication in constructing the exquisite drawings in this atlas are best noted in the meticulous details of the illustrations themselves.

I would also like to express my sincere thanks to Dr. Andrew Rauscher for his review and suggestions on the manuscript.

Jordan Katz, M.D.

Introduction

Scope

This text is designed to provide the physician with an atlas of nerve block techniques in as simple and straightforward a manner as possible. Almost all clinically useful procedures are included. By following the written instructions and referring to the appropriate illustrations, the clinician should be able to perform successful nerve block analgesia.

Indications for Nerve Blocks

Indications fall into two general catagories—diagnostic and therapeutic. The assumption has been made that the physician doing the block has thoroughly evaluated the clinical situation and determined a need for a particular block procedure for diagnosis or therapy.

Preparation of the Patient

It is just as important to adequately prepare the patient for a nerve block as it is for any other invasive technique. Physiologically, the patient should be in optimal condition, especially if major nerve block procedures are contemplated. Of similar importance is the psychological preparation of the patient. This should include a brief discussion on why the procedure is being done, as well as how it is to be accomplished. Patient cooperation is often essential.

If a paresthesia is to be sought, the patient should be aware of where and what he or she will feel. This has the dual purpose of promoting patient cooperation and assisting the practitioner in ascertaining if a "true" response has been obtained. Mild sedation in the form of tranquilizing and/or narcotic drugs is usually helpful, especially in the more difficult or painful blocks, such as the sciatic nerve block.

The area to be blocked should be adequately prepped and draped. Patient positioning for the majority of nerve blocking techniques is described. In some instances the position is so obvious that there is no need to further delineate it. It should be noted that variations in the patient's anatomy or other unusual circumstances, such as pain, may necessitate modification of the position recommended in the text.

Technique

The technique described for each block is one the author has found reliable in producing the desired results. This does not imply that other techniques cannot be used successfully. The aficionado in this specialized area of medicine often can perform any one block using a variety of techniques. This text was designed specifically for the clinician who does not have this far-ranging experience.

For the most part a single technique is described. For certain blocks, however, such as sciatic nerve or brachial plexus blocks, several techniques are illustrated. The choice of a particular technique when more than one is described is based on specific indications or clinician preference. To illustrate a specific indication, the axillary approach to the brachial plexus would probably be more ideal for procedures below the level of the elbow, and obviously could not be used for interventions in the upper arm or shoulder, while the interscalene technique provides adequate anesthesia for shoulder and upper arm procedures.

The needle gauge and length have been determined for average-size patients with usual anatomy. For infiltration procedures, long beveled needles should be used; for nerve block procedures, short beveled needles are preferred. The usual depth from skin to nerve is given for most procedures. This depth is based on average anatomic features and may have to be modified in the individual patient. Obviously, the thin, emaciated, extremely muscular, or obese might fall outside the ranges stated.

Local Anesthetics

Local anesthetic dosages are presented either as dilute solutions, usual solutions, or concentrated solutions. In general, dilute solutions are used for infiltration-type procedures, whereas the usual concentrations are for major nerve blocks. When the nerve is particularly large (e.g., sciatic nerve), a concentrated local anesthetic solution is recommended. The volume of local anesthetic recommended herein is for the average patient in good health. Variations based on physical condition, age of patient, etc., may have to occur. In Table 1 the common local anesthetics used for infiltration or nerve block procedures are listed and comparable concentrations noted.

Allergic or anaphylactic reactions to local anesthetics are extremely rare. However, local anesthetic reactions due to excess dosage, inadvertent intravascular placement, or rapid absorption from highly vascular areas are not infrequent. The basic principles for prevention of local anesthetic reaction are not to exceed the recommended volume and concentration of the local anesthetic being injected, aspirate before injection of any large volume of local anesthetic, and look for and recognize premonitory signs of overdose. Excess premedication should be avoided since verbal contact with the patient is of utmost importance. It is beyond the scope of this book to go into the therapy of local anesthetic overdose. The reader is referred to any standard text for details.

Neurolytics

The use of neurolytic agents is mentioned in the text for certain nerve block procedures, such as lumbar sympathetic block. It is not the purpose of this atlas to discuss the pros and cons of neurolytic agents or the concentrations and amounts to be used for any specific procedure. The few instances when neurolytics are mentioned are just to inform the reader that neurolytic techniques are used with the nerve block procedure described when long term effects are necessary.

Aids to Nerve Blockade

The basic premise of this book is to present in the simplest format a technique to block any given nerve. In several instances the text mentions that certain aids may be useful when

TABLE 1

| Drug | Concentration (%) | | |
	Dilute	Usual	Concentrated
Procaine	0.5	1.0	1.0–2.0
Chloroprocaine	0.25–0.5	1.0–2.0	2.0
Lidocaine	0.25–0.5	1.0–1.5	1.5–2.0
Mepivacaine	0.25–0.5	1.0–1.5	1.5–2.0
Prilocaine	0.5–1.0	1.0–2.0	2.0–3.0
Tetracaine		0.1–0.15	0.15–0.2
Bupivacaine	0.125–0.25	0.25–0.5	0.5
Etidocaine	0.25–0.5	0.5–1.0	1.0–1.5

Note: If a vasoconstrictor is to be used, adrenaline 1:200,000 is the preferred additive.

attempting a more difficult procedure, such as a celiac plexus block. In essence there are two types of devices that can be used—nerve stimulators and fluoroscopy.

Most nerve stimulators are similar in design. Their purpose is to transmit an electrical stimulus from the tip of the blocking needle, now acting as a needle electrode, causing an evoked response in the form of a muscle twitch. By reducing the strength of the stimulus and maintaining an evoked response, the needle gradually approaches the nerve. The local anesthetic solution is then injected.

Fluoroscopy is also a useful aid, especially when deeper nerves are sought. The position of the needle in relation to bony landmarks can be observed. Radiopaque substance, when used, will show the direction of spread of local anesthetic or neurolytic solutions. The incorporation of fluoroscopy and nerve stimulators into nerve blocking procedures is useful, even in the most experienced hands, when dealing with the more technically difficult nerve block situations.

Atlas of Regional Anesthesia

Head

Scalp

Anatomy

From the nose to the occiput, the skin overlying the skull is innervated by (1) the supratrochlear and supraorbital branches of the ophthalmic division of the trigeminal nerve, (2) the zygomaticotemporal and zygomaticofacial branches of the maxillary division, (3) the auriculotemporal branch arising from the mandibular division, and (4) the lesser and greater occipital nerves from C2 and C3.

Technique

A subcutaneous infiltration is made just above the nose, over the eyebrows to the outer aspect of the orbit bilaterally. This infiltration is continued so that a wheal will be raised just above the ear and further posteriorly, meeting at the midline of the occiput. As the needle is advanced above the periosteum, local anesthetic should be continuously injected. Greater amounts of local anesthetic should be deposited in the areas of the supraorbital, auriculotemporal, and greater and lesser occipital nerves. The peripheral branches of these nerves course between the skin and the periosteum. A dilute local anesthetic solution mixed with epinephrine 1:200,000 should be used. Large volumes will be required to completely anesthetize the scalp.

An alternate technique for limited procedures on the scalp is accomplished by depositing local anesthetic in a triangular configuration around the lesion.

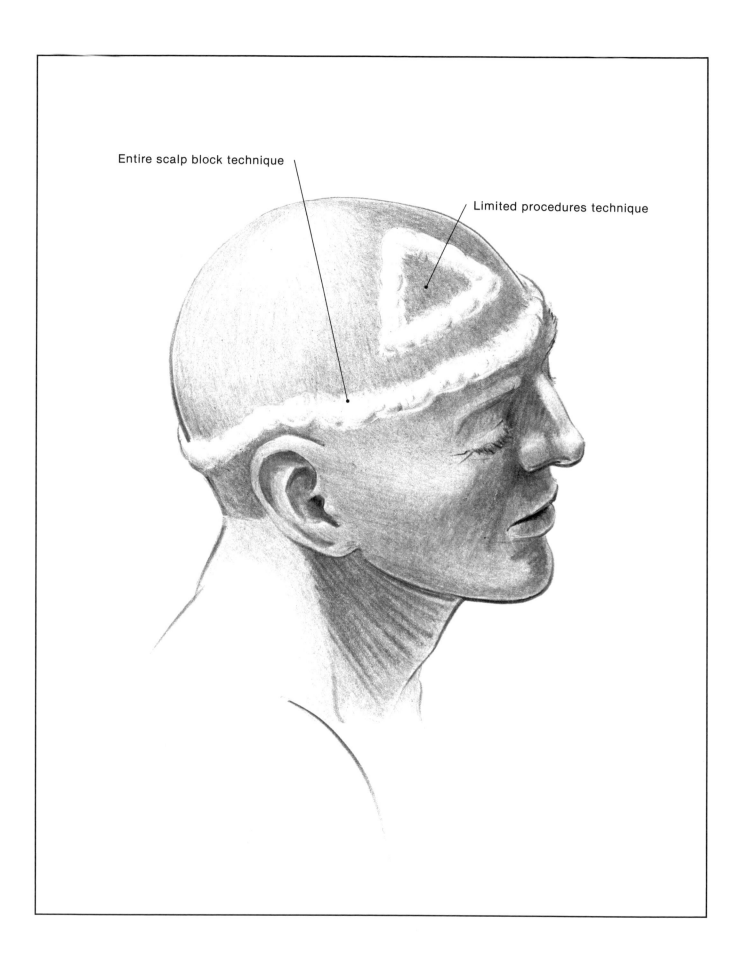

Entire scalp block technique

Limited procedures technique

Gasserian Ganglion

Anatomy

The gasserian ganglion (trigeminal ganglion, semilunar ganglion) is formed from two roots starting along the ventral surface of the brainstem at the midpontine level. The roots pass forward and laterally within the posterior cranial fossa across the superior border of the petrous temporal bone. They enter a recess called Meckel's cave (trigeminal cave) which is formed by an invagination of the dura mater of the posterior cranial fossa. In this recess lies the crescent shaped ganglion of the trigeminal nerve, from whose anterior convex border arise the ophthalmic, maxillary, and mandibular divisions of the nerve.

Technique

This block should be performed with radiologic confirmation of needle position. The patient lies in the neutral position with head slightly extended. The length of the zygomatic arch is noted and its midpoint marked. Approximately 1 inch (depending on the width of the face) lateral to the corner of the mouth, on the involved side and slightly superiorly (opposite the upper second molar), a skin wheal is raised. A 4-inch, 22-gauge needle with stylet in place is inserted so that it will pass through the substance of the cheek, travelling just medial to the ramus of the mandible in a cephalad and mediad direction toward the pupil of the eye. When viewed from the front the needle should point to the pupil of the eye; when viewed from the side it should be directed deep to the mark on the midpoint of the zygomatic arch. The needle tip should then encounter the base of the skull at a point somewhat anterior to the foramen ovale. This should be verified radiologically. The needle is then redirected posteriorly until the foramen is entered. As the needle approaches the foramen, paresthesias of the mandibular nerve may be encountered. If this is the case, the needle should be repositioned until it enters the foramen without stimulating the mandibular nerve, again under radiologic guidance. After careful aspiration for blood and cerebral spinal fluid, 1 to 3 cc of local anesthetic is injected slowly until the desired clinical effect occurs.

Note: Since an invagination of the dura surrounds the posterior two-thirds of the ganglion (see above) and is in direct continuity with the cerebrospinal fluid (CSF) within the brain, even a very small amount of local anesthetic injected there could cause unconsciousness and cardiorespiratory arrest. The use of neurolytic agents for the procedure described above should be avoided. Specialized techniques for retrogasserian injection have been developed using very precise stereotaxic approaches. This block should be done under controlled conditions and by experienced personnel only.

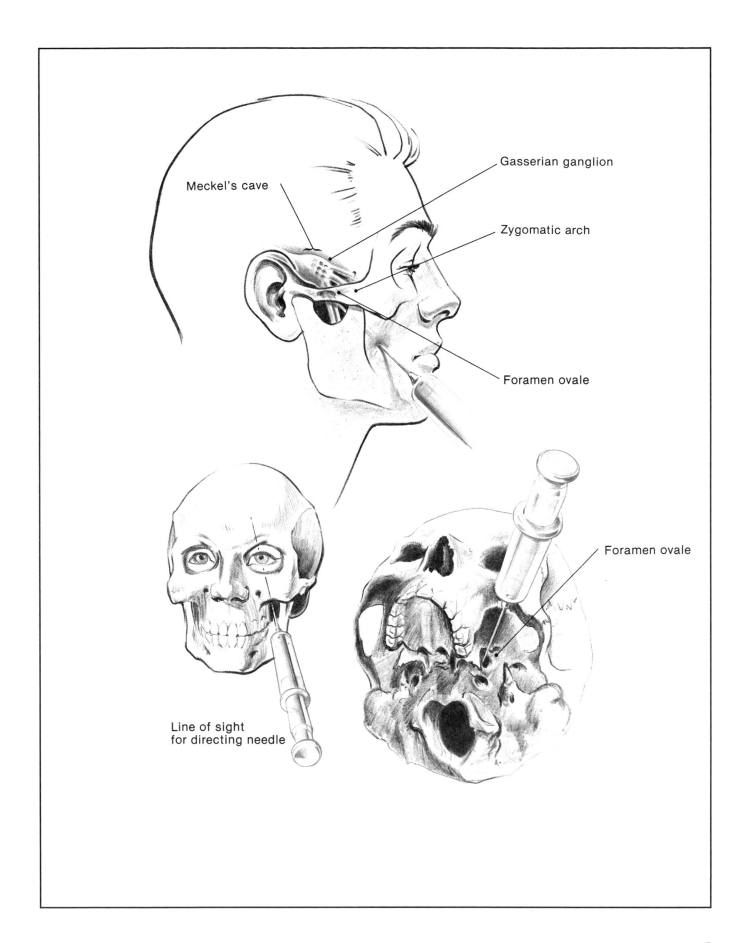

Meckel's cave

Gasserian ganglion

Zygomatic arch

Foramen ovale

Foramen ovale

Line of sight
for directing needle

Nasociliary, Long Ciliary, and Anterior Ethmoidal Nerves

Anatomy

The ophthalmic nerve is the smallest of the three divisions of trigeminal ganglion. It runs forward from the medial surface of the ganglion via the cavernous sinus and after dividing into the three main branches—the nasociliary, frontal, and lacrimal nerves—passes into the orbit through the superior orbital fissure. There are no indications for blocking the ophthalmic nerve per se and therefore only its peripheral branches will be considered. After entering the orbit the nasociliary nerve reaches the medial wall, where it exits via the anterior ethmoid foramen and eventually terminates in the nasal cavity. In its course it gives off several branches, the long ciliary and infratrochlear nerves, and terminates as the anterior ethmoidal nerve.

Technique

The patient lies supine, eyes directed forward. At the innermost aspect of the orbit (approximately ½ inch above the inner canthus) a 2-inch, 25-gauge needle is inserted. The needle follows the nasal wall of the orbit for about 1 inch. One to two cubic centimeters of local anesthetic is deposited at this point and additional small quantities are infiltrated as the needle is withdrawn to the skin.

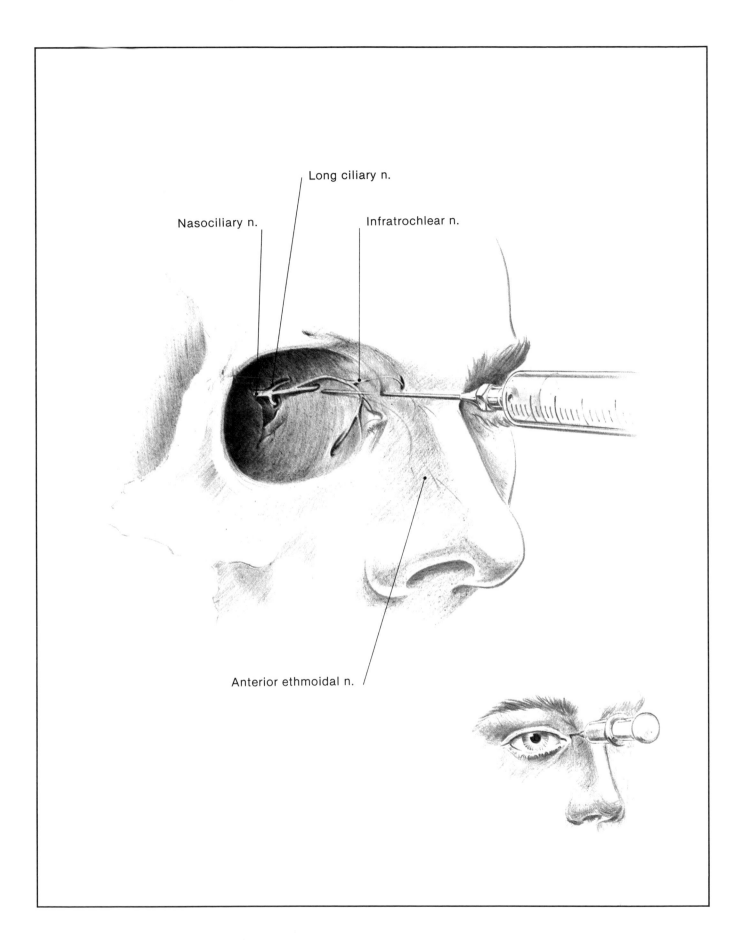

Long ciliary n.

Nasociliary n.

Infratrochlear n.

Anterior ethmoidal n.

Supraorbital Nerve

Anatomy

The frontal nerve, largest branch of the ophthalmic nerve, enters the orbit via the superior orbital fissure and runs forward beneath the periosteum of the orbital roof, dividing into a larger lateral supraorbital nerve and a smaller medial supratrochlear nerve. These branches leave the orbital cavity anteriorly and distribute fibers to the upper eyelids, forehead and anterior part of the scalp, with the supraorbital nerve extending fibers that reach as far back as the vertex of the cranium.

Technique

The patient lies supine with head in neutral position. The supraorbital notch is easily palpated in the middle of the upper eyebrow and is usually in a direct line with the pupil of the eye. A ½-inch, 25-gauge needle is inserted aiming directly at the notch. Usually a paresthesia is elicited before the bone is contacted. If, however, the bone is contacted first, the direction of the needle should be moved slightly in a fanlike distribution. After eliciting a paresthesia, 2 to 3 cc of local anesthetic is injected. If no distinct paresthesia can be obtained, 3 cc of local anesthetic is distributed in the vicinity of the notch.

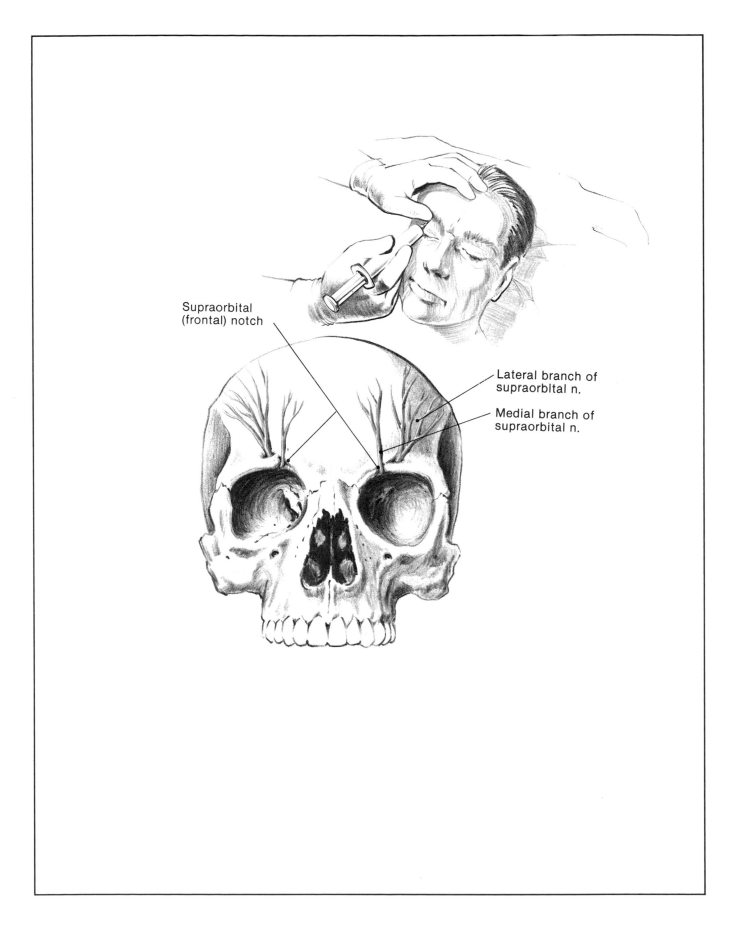

Supraorbital
(frontal) notch

Lateral branch of
supraorbital n.

Medial branch of
supraorbital n.

Supratrochlear Nerve

Anatomy

See anatomy of supraorbital nerve (p. 8).

Technique

Patient lies supine with head in the neutral position. A ½-inch, 25-gauge needle is inserted at the point where the bridge of the nose meets the supraorbital ridge. A paresthesia is usually elicited as the needle is advanced into the soft tissue. Two cubic centimeters of local anesthetic is then injected. If a paresthesia to the middle of the forehead is not easily obtained, soft tissue infiltration of 2 to 3 cc of local anesthetic will block the nerve.

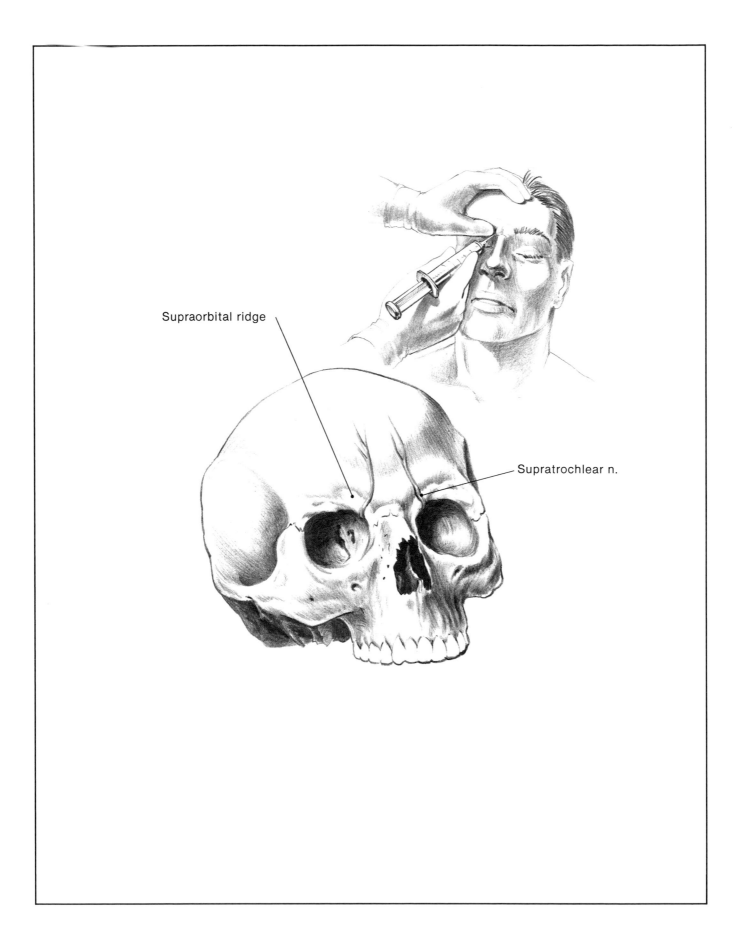

Supraorbital ridge

Supratrochlear n.

Maxillary Nerve

Anatomy

The maxillary nerve leaves the gasserian ganglion and proceeds horizontally and forward along the inferior lateral border of the cavernous sinus. It exits the middle cranial fossa through the foramen rotundum and enters the pterygopalatine fossa, where its major branches arise.

Technique

The patient lies supine, head turned so that the side to be blocked is uppermost. The zygomatic arch is palpated, as is the notch of the mandible. The patient is asked to open his mouth slightly. A 3-inch, 22-gauge block needle is inserted just beneath the zygomatic arch at approximately the midpoint of the notch of the mandible. The needle is advanced 1½ to 2 inches perpendicular to the base of the skull until the lateral pterygoid plate is encountered. This depth should be noted. The needle is then withdrawn to the subcutaneous tissue and reinserted so as to slip past the anterior margin of the lateral pterygoid plate (in the general direction of the eye). Approximately ½ inch deeper than when the plate was first touched, paresthesias of the mandibular nerve should be elicited. This is usually felt by the patient in the upper jaw. Three to five cubic centimeters of local anesthetic is injected after careful aspiration.

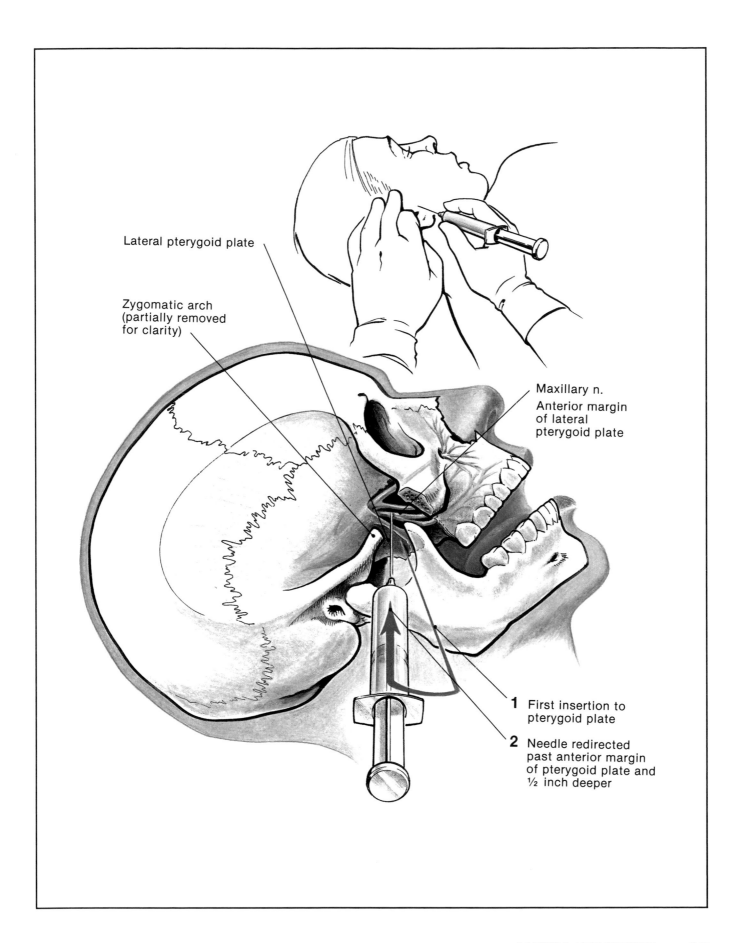

Lateral pterygoid plate

Zygomatic arch
(partially removed
for clarity)

Maxillary n.

Anterior margin
of lateral
pterygoid plate

1 First insertion to
pterygoid plate

2 Needle redirected
past anterior margin
of pterygoid plate and
½ inch deeper

Infraorbital Nerve

Anatomy

The infraorbital nerve is the main continuation and largest terminal branch of the maxillary nerve. It enters the orbit of the eye through the infraorbital fissure, and lies on the floor of the orbit in the infraorbital groove. It emerges from the orbit onto the face via the infraorbital foramen. There it sends out terminal cutaneous branches that innervate the lower eyelid, upper lip, and side of the nose. Sensation to the upper incisor and canine teeth and gingiva is provided by the anterior superior alveolar branch.

Technique

The patient lies supine, head in the neutral position. The infraorbital foramen is easily palpated on the infraorbital ridge just below the pupil of the eye, on a line between the pupil and the corner of the lips. The foramen is approached from a point ½ inch below and slightly medial to it with a ½-inch, 25-gauge needle. A paresthesia to the upper lip is often obtained and the local anesthetic is injected at that time. If paresthesia does not occur, 2 to 3 cc of local anesthetic is deposited over the area of the palpated foramen.

Note: The foramen can also be approached from the lateral aspect and the needle can actually be inserted into the canal. This may cause direct nerve trauma, however, and this approach is not advised for routine local anesthetic infiltration.

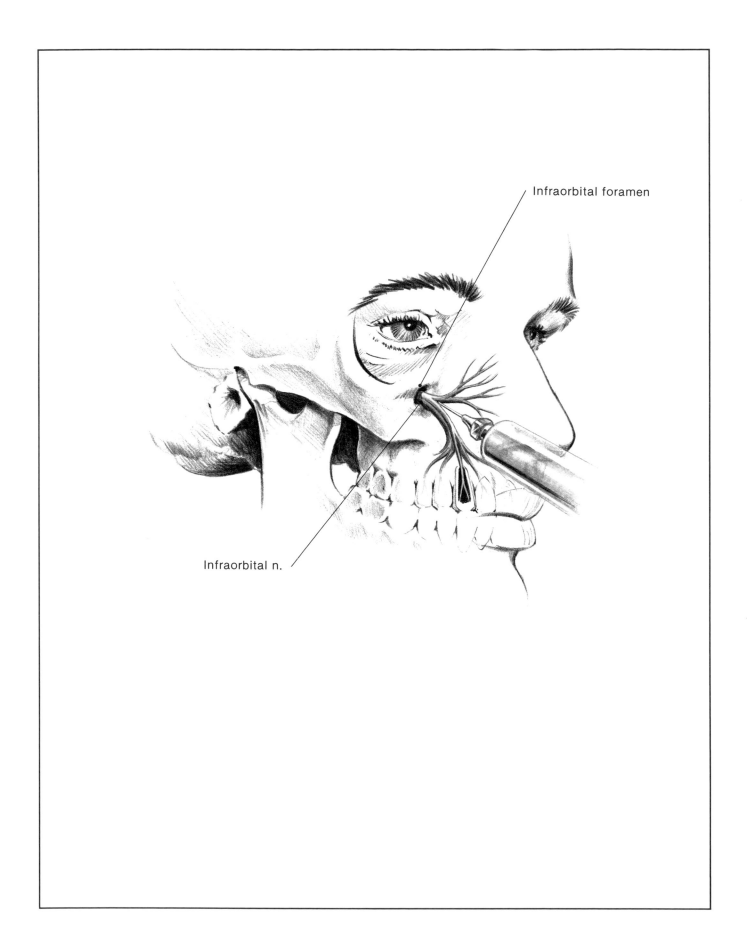

Infraorbital foramen

Infraorbital n.

Sphenopalatine Ganglion

Anatomy

The sphenopalatine (pterygopalatine) ganglia is a small triangular structure lying in the pterygopalatine fossa. It receives sensory roots from the maxillary nerve, a motor root via the greater superficial petrosal nerve (a branch of the facial nerve), and a sympathetic root from the carotid plexus through the deep petrosal nerve. Coming from the ganglia are many small branches, including an orbital branch that innervates the periosteum of the orbit and lacrimal gland, a nasal branch that includes the posterior superior nasal and nasal palatine nerves that supply the gums, hard palate, soft palate, uvula, and part of the tonsils.

Technique

The patient is positioned supine with a pillow under the shoulders and mouth wide open. A 120 degree angle needle with a fine tip is required. The greater palatine foramen is located at the posterior portion of the hard palate just medial to the gumline opposite the third molar. The angled needle is advanced 1½ to 2 inches through the foramen in a superior and slightly posterior direction. The maxillary nerve is immediately above the ganglia. Paresthesia may be elicited. Two cubic centimeters of local anesthetic solution is injected after which the sphenopalatine ganglion (perhaps the maxillary nerve as well) will be blocked. This injection will anesthetize the posterior palatine, middle palatine, anterior palatine, and nasal palatine nerves. It may also anesthetize other peripheral branches of the maxillary nerve.

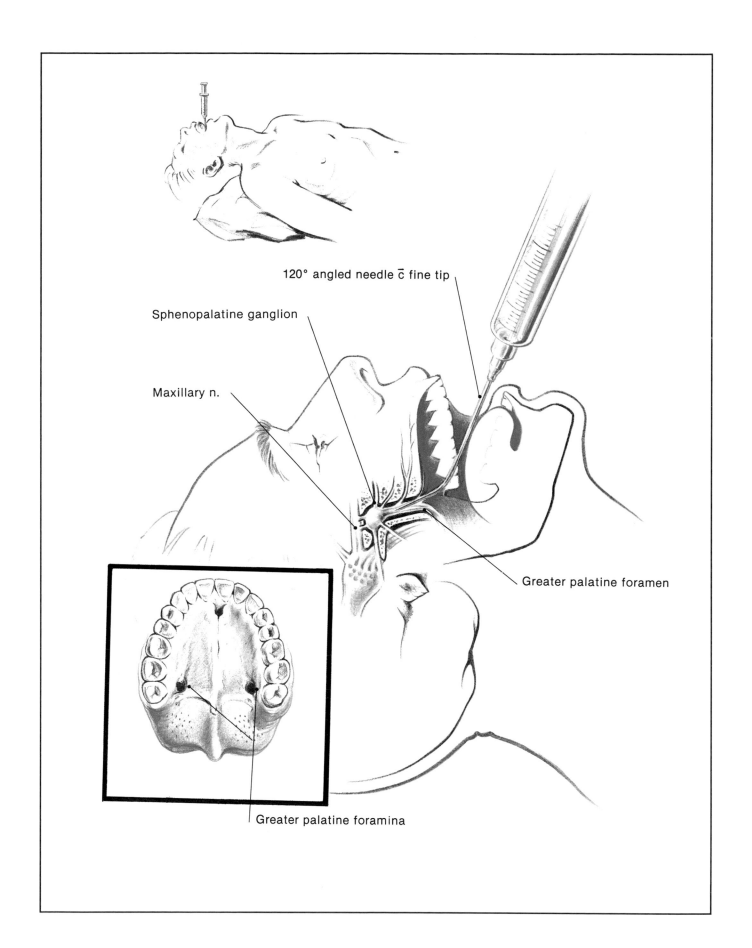

120° angled needle c̄ fine tip

Sphenopalatine ganglion

Maxillary n.

Greater palatine foramen

Greater palatine foramina

Mandibular Nerve

Anatomy

The mandibular nerve, third and largest division of the trigeminal nerve, is formed by the fusion of a slender motor root with the larger inferior branch from the trigeminal ganglion. These nerve bundles leave the cranial cavity through the foramen ovale and send branches to the dura mater and the medial pterygoid, tensor tympani, and tensor palatine muscles. Just below the foramen the mandibular trunk divides into smaller anterior and larger posterior divisions. The anterior division provides fibers to the muscles of mastication (lateral pterygoid, temporalis, and masseter muscles). It also has some sensory fibers that go to the skin in the region of the angle of the mouth via the long buccal nerve. The posterior division is mostly sensory and rapidly divides into the inferior alveolar, lingual, and auriculotemporal nerves.

Technique

The patient lies supine, head turned to the side. The zygomatic arch is palpated, as is the notch of the ramus of the mandible. The patient is asked to open the mouth slightly. A 3-inch, 22-gauge block needle is inserted just beneath the zygomatic arch approximately at the midpoint of the notch of the mandible. The needle is advanced for 1½ to 2 inches perpendicular to the base of the skull. The lateral pterygoid plate should then be encountered. The needle is then withdrawn to the subcutaneous tissue and directed posteriorly to the plate in the general direction of the ear. About ½ inch beyond the pterygoid plate a paresthesia to the lower jaw or tongue will indicate that the mandibular nerve has been contacted. Five to eight cubic centimeters of solution is injected.

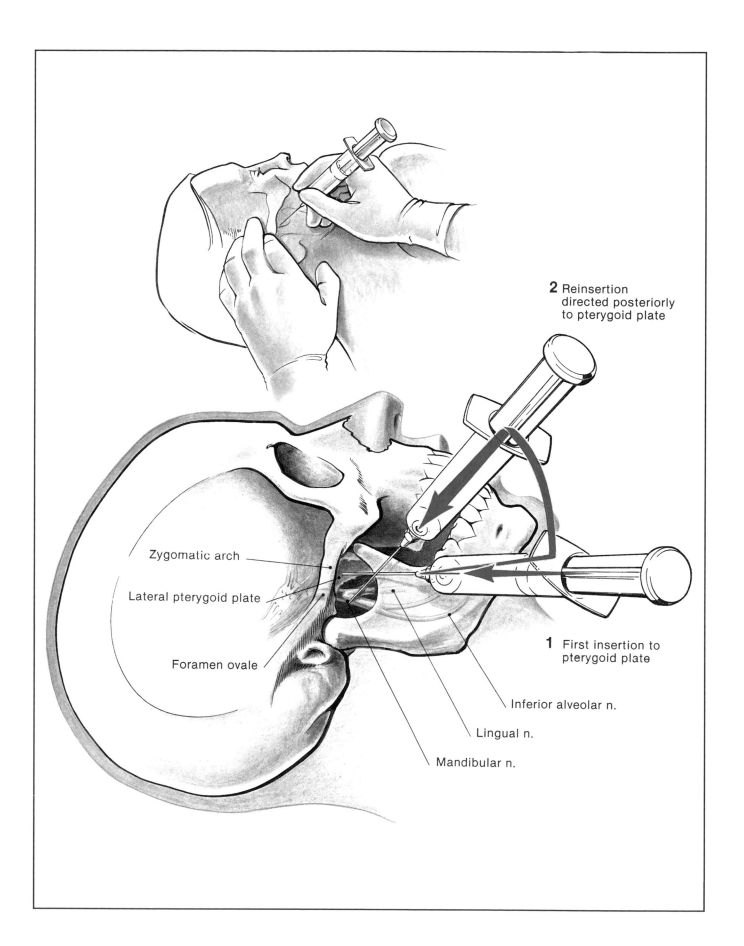

2 Reinsertion
directed posteriorly
to pterygoid plate

1 First insertion to
pterygoid plate

Zygomatic arch

Lateral pterygoid plate

Foramen ovale

Inferior alveolar n.

Lingual n.

Mandibular n.

Inferior Alveolar and Lingual Nerves

Anatomy

The inferior alveolar nerve is the largest branch of the mandibular nerve. From its origin it passes downward behind the lingual nerve on the medial surface of the mandible to enter the mandibular canal. It then passes forward in the substance of the mandible, distributing branches to the lower molar and premolar teeth and adjacent parts of the gingiva. Near the mental foramen it divides into the incisor branch, which continues forward in the mandible to supply the canine and incisor teeth, and the larger mental branch, which passes out of its bony canal via the mental foramen.

The lingual nerve passes downward and forward anterior to the inferior alveolar nerve, along the medial aspect of the ramus of the mandible on its way toward its termination in the tongue. It is joined by branches of the chorda tympani. Major sensory innervation is to the mucosa of the anterior two-thirds of the tongue. The fibers of the chorda tympani that accompany it subserve taste in the anterior two-thirds of the tongue, with the exception of the circumvallate papillae. The lingual nerve also supplies secretory fibers to the submandibular and sublingual salivary glands.

Technique

Since the same procedure is used for the block of both nerves, a single description will suffice. The patient lies in the neutral position with mouth wide open. The anterior border of the ramus of the mandible is palpated just above the last molar of the lower jaw. A 2-inch block needle is inserted above the palpating finger and between the mucosa and inner surface of the ramus of the mandible. Local anesthetic is infiltrated slowly as the needle is advanced posteriorly and slightly superiorly along the inner surface of the ramus to a depth of approximately 1 to 1½ inches. If a paresthesia to the teeth or anterior portion of the tongue has not been elicited by the advancing needle, an additional 5 cc of local anesthetic is infiltrated as the needle is slowly withdrawn.

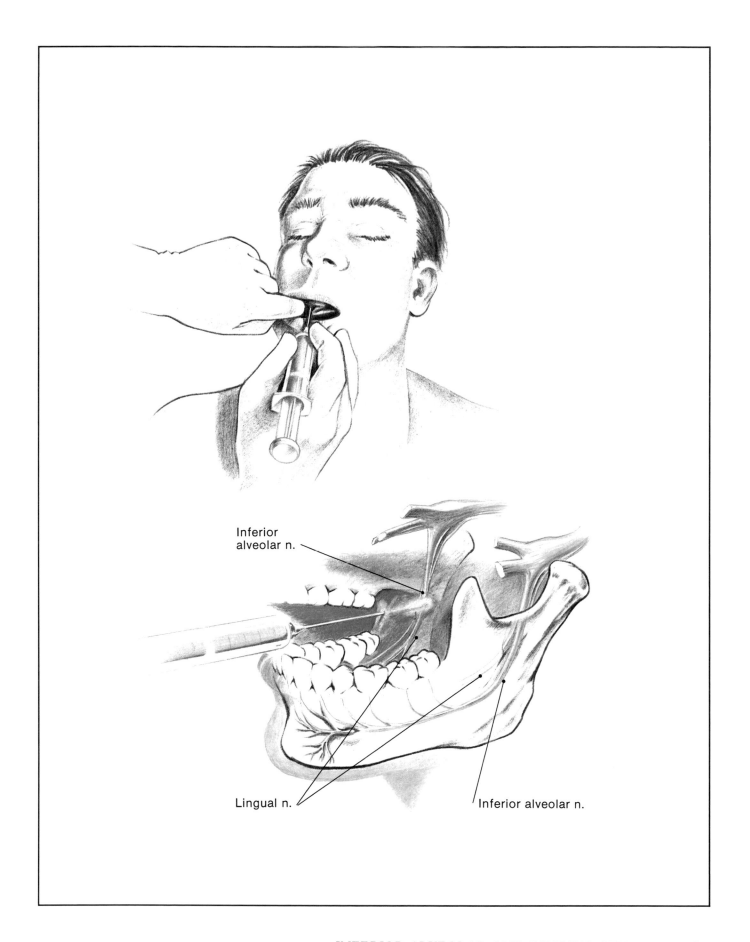

Inferior
alveolar n.

Lingual n.

Inferior alveolar n.

Auriculotemporal Nerve

Anatomy

This nerve arises from the posterior root of the mandibular nerve and passes through the substance of the parotid gland between the external auditory meatus and the temporomandibular joint. Finally, it ascends over the zygomatic arch accompanying the superficial temporal artery. It supplies the skin of the temporal region and lateral part of the scalp. In its course it gives off small nerve twigs to the external auditory meatus, tympanic membrane, portions of the pinna, and the temporomandibular joint.

Technique

A ½-inch, 25-gauge block needle is inserted in front of the ear at the origin of the zygoma. The temporal artery can be palpated in this area. Three cubic centimeters of local anesthetic are infiltrated in the skin down to the root of the zygomatic arch. This block will also numb the nerve's peripheral branches—the anterior auricular, superficial temporal, and tympanic nerves.

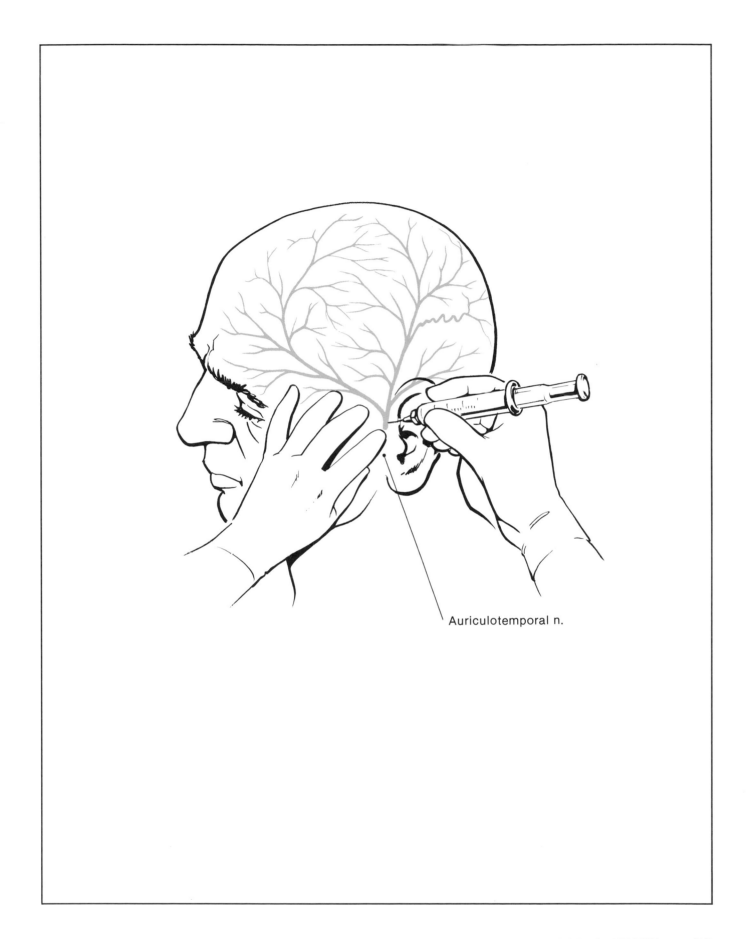

Auriculotemporal n.

Long Buccal Nerve

Anatomy

The long buccal nerve is a branch of the anterior division of the mandibular nerve. It innervates the skin at the angle of the mouth and the corresponding mucous membrane inside the cheek.

Technique

The patient's head is in the neutral position. The terminal branches of the long buccal nerve are usually blocked by inserting a ½-inch, 25-gauge needle at the commissure of the lips. Infiltration of 1 to 2 cc of local anesthetic as the needle is passed subcutaneously from the commissure toward the cheek will block the nerves.

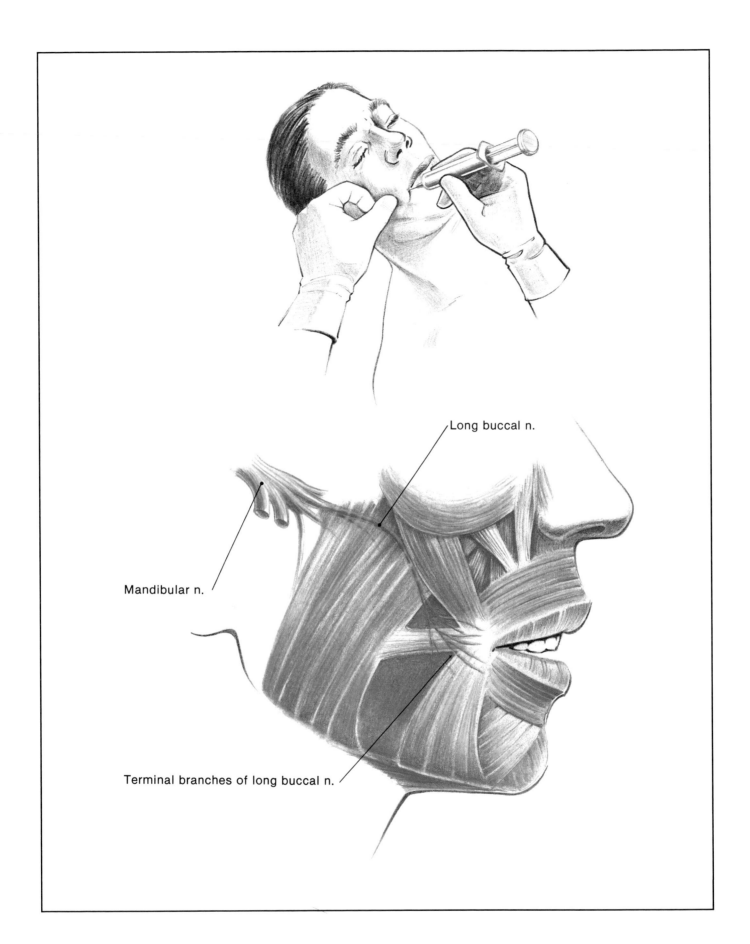

Long buccal n.

Mandibular n.

Terminal branches of long buccal n.

Masseter Nerve

Anatomy

Immediately after the mandibular nerve divides into its major inferior alveolar and lingual divisions, the masseter nerve branches off from the former. The masseter nerve is the motor nerve to the masseter muscle.

Technique

The masseter nerve is blocked during infiltration of the mandibular nerve (p. 18) and block of the inferior alveolar nerve (p. 20). There is no procedure specific to the masseter nerve.

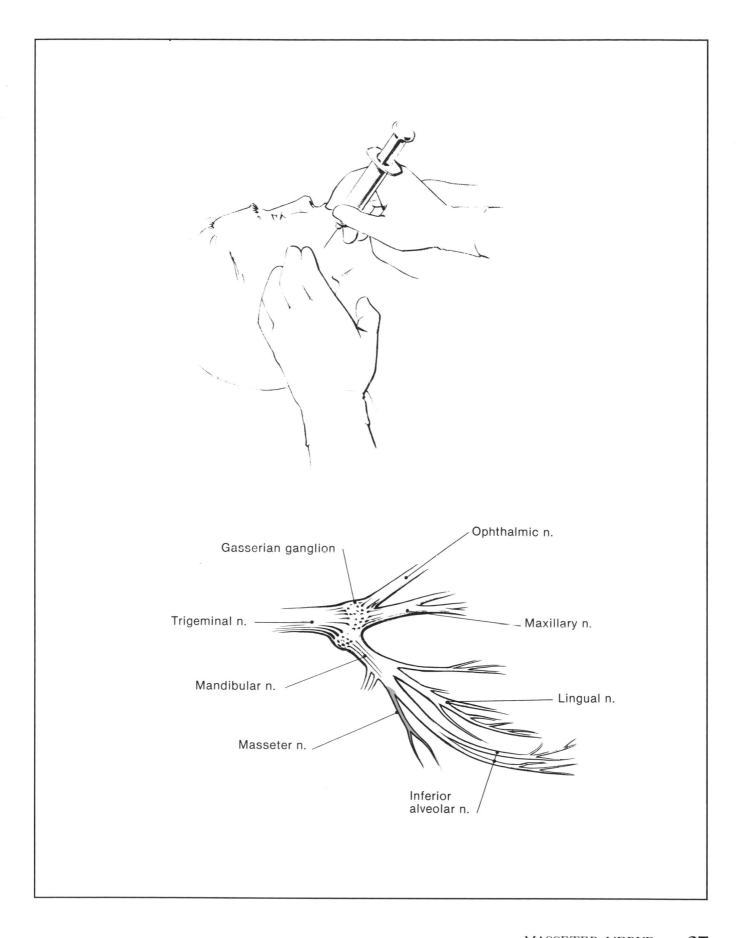

Gasserian ganglion

Ophthalmic n.

Trigeminal n.

Maxillary n.

Mandibular n.

Lingual n.

Masseter n.

Inferior
alveolar n.

Mental Nerve

Anatomy

The mental nerve is one of the two terminal branches of the inferior alveolar nerve. It emerges via the mental canal. This causes it to make an acute turn, since the canal angles posteriorly and superiorly from its origin deep within the mandible to its terminus at the mental foramen. The mental nerve innervates the lower lip and corresponding gingival surface from the corner of the mouth to the midline.

Technique

With the patient lying supine, head in the midline, the mental foramen is palpated, usually in the middle of the mandible just below the first premolar tooth or corner of the mouth. The foramen is approached anteriorly with a ½- to 1-inch, 23-gauge needle. The mandible is contacted and the needle advanced until the foramen is identified as a depression on the bone. A paresthesia may or may not be elicited. Three cubic centimeters of local anesthetic is injected.

Note: The nerve may also be approached posteriorly with the tip of the needle searching for and entering the opening of the mental canal. This technique may cause impingement on the nerve, however, and is not recommended for routine blocks.

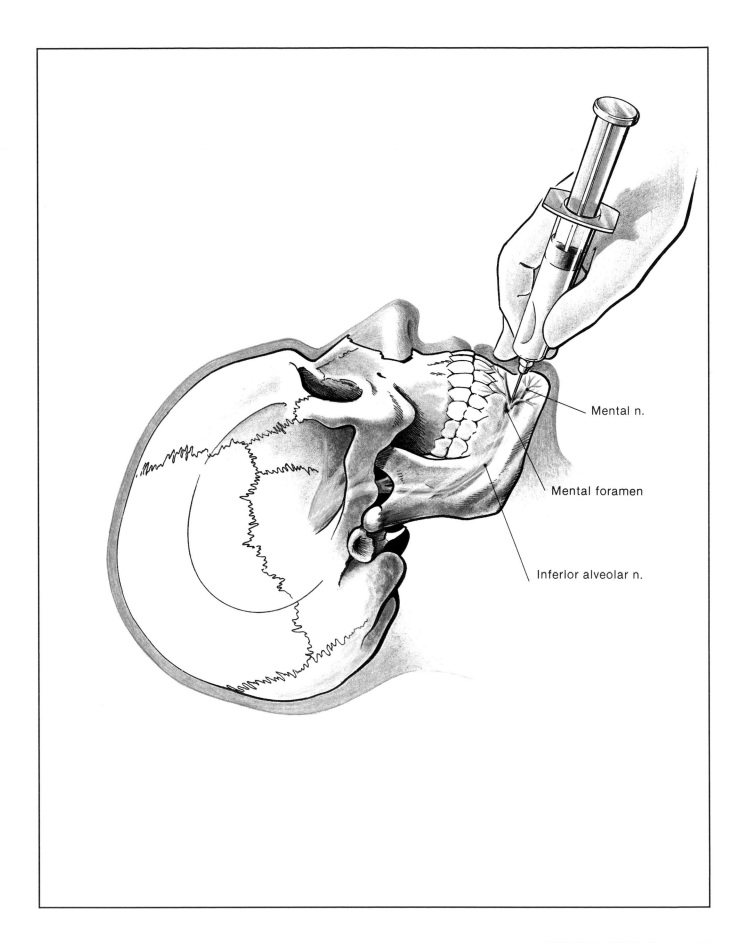

Mental n.

Mental foramen

Inferior alveolar n.

Eye

Anatomy

Major autonomic innervation of the eye is via the ciliary ganglion that lies in the posterior portion of the orbit between the optic nerve and lateral rectus muscle. The eye gets parasympathetic innervation from the inferior branch of the oculomotor nerve. It gets sympathetic sensation from fibers whose cell bodies originate in the superior cervical ganglion, the axons of which course through the carotid and cavernous plexi. A sensory root is composed of fibers from the ophthalmic nerve. Emerging from the ciliary ganglion are multiple slender rami distributed to the ciliary body, the muscles of the iris, and the extrinsic muscles. The lateral rectus muscle is innervated by a branch of the sixth cranial nerve, the superior oblique by the fourth cranial nerve, and all the other extrinsic muscles by branches of the third cranial (oculomotor) nerve. Vision is transmitted via the optic nerve.

Technique

The patient lies supine, face in the neutral position. Patient is told to look upward, backward, and slightly inward. The lower lateral aspect of the orbit is palpated, and at its most inferior point a 3.5-cm, 25-gauge needle is inserted through the lid and toward the apex of the orbit. The needle length is critical in order that vessels at the apex of the orbit are not punctured. Small amounts of local anesthetic (less than 1 cc) should be infiltrated as the needle is advanced between the globe and the bony wall of the orbit. The needle should advance without meeting any undue resistance. There will be minor "pops" as the needle passes through first the orbital septum and then the muscle cone. If significant resistance is met, the needle has encountered either a muscle, the globe, or the wall of the orbit and should be redirected. When the needle is inserted to its full depth of 3.5 cm, 2 to 3 cc of local anesthetic

(for the majority of ophthalmologic procedures) is injected slowly after careful aspiration. For certain procedures, such as enucleation, 4 cc or more of local anesthetic may be required. The needle is withdrawn and the patient told to look straight ahead. The lids are closed. The globe is then gently massaged intermittently for several minutes. Within 5 minutes after injection surgery may be started.

Note: Several short-bevel needles that are precisely 3.5 cm from hub to tip are used for this procedure. A slight proptosis will usually be noted after injection, but this dissipates rapidly. Retrobulbar hemorrhage is an unlikely complication, but it should be looked for. It is noted by proptosis, firmness of the globe, and discoloration, usually in the lower fornix but at times elsewhere around the eyeball. If retrobulbar hemorrhage is to occur, it will be noted within 5 minutes.

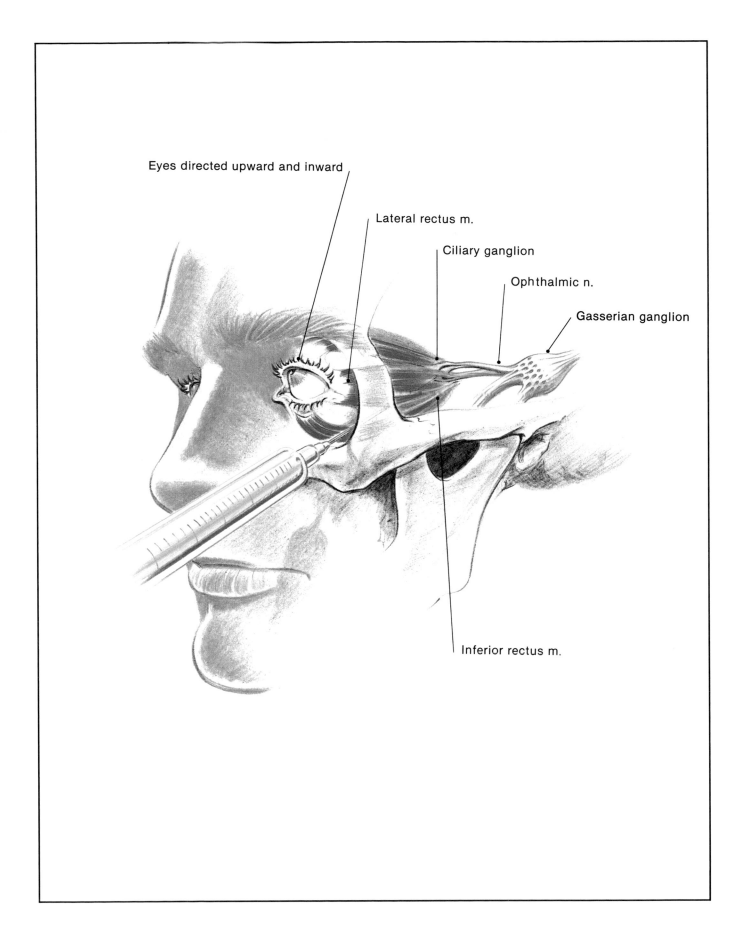

Eyes directed upward and inward

Lateral rectus m.

Ciliary ganglion

Ophthalmic n.

Gasserian ganglion

Inferior rectus m.

Facial Nerve

Anatomy

The facial nerve has two roots—motor and sensory. The latter is called the nervus intermedius. The facial nerve arises from the brainstem at the low border of the pons. From there both roots travel together across the subarachnoid space to enter the internal auditory meatus. After passing through the petrous temporal bone it exits the skull at the stylomastoid foramen. It then passes downward and forward, lateral to the styloid process, to eventually enter into and traverse the parotid gland. There it divides into its terminal branches. These branches innervate the muscles that provide facial expression. Prior to entering the parotid, several smaller branches are given off, including those to the stylohyoid, digastric, and stapedius muscles, the chorda tympani, and the posterior auricular nerve.

Technique

The patient lies supine, head turned away from the side to be injected. A skin wheal is made over the anterior edge of the mastoid process, approximately opposite the midpoint of ramus of the mandible and immediately below the external auditory meatus. A 1-inch, 23-gauge block needle is inserted until it contacts the anterior edge of the mastoid process. It is then directed to slide past the bone and advanced about ½ inch deeper. This should place the tip of the needle just below the stylomastoid foramen, where 3 cc of local anesthetic is injected.

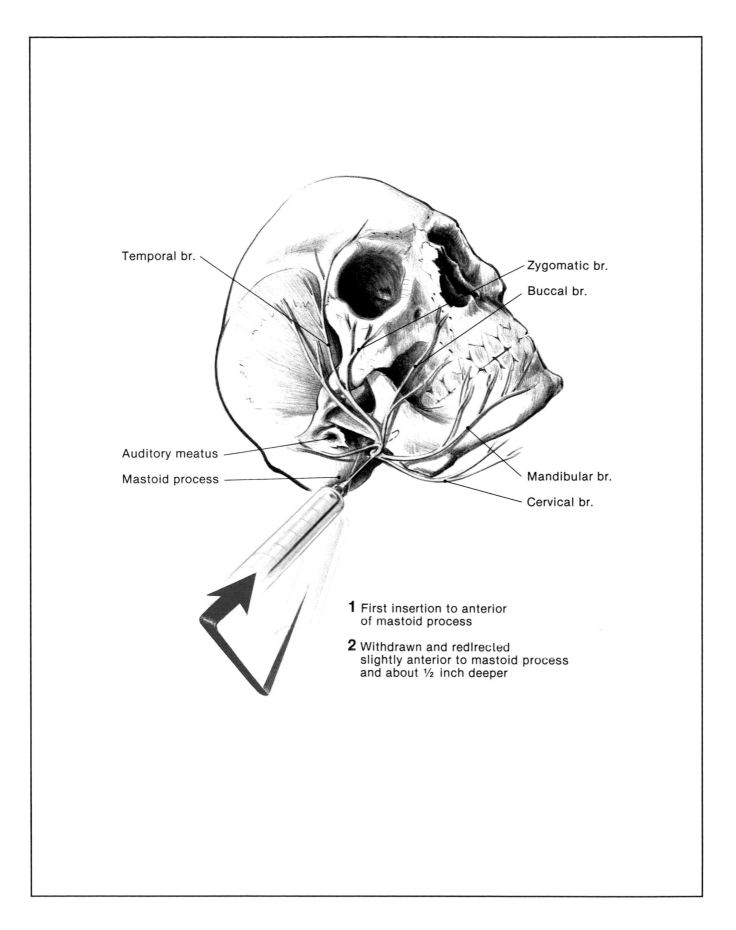

Temporal br.

Zygomatic br.

Buccal br.

Auditory meatus

Mastoid process

Mandibular br.

Cervical br.

1 First insertion to anterior
of mastoid process

2 Withdrawn and redirected
slightly anterior to mastoid process
and about ½ inch deeper

Nose

Anatomy

The nose has a complex innervation, with the skin, lateral wall, and septum each having independent nerve supplies. The lateral wall is innervated by the anterior ethmoidal nerve, multiple branches of the olfactory nerves, and terminal branches emanating from the sphenopalatine ganglion. The septum is innervated posteriorly by branches of the sphenopalatine nerve and anteriorly by the anterior ethmoidal nerve. Branches of the supratrochlear, nasociliary, and infraorbital nerves are involved in providing sensation to the skin of the nose.

Technique

The mucous membranes of the nose are best anesthetized with topical anesthesia using 4% cocaine (or a local anesthetic with good surface anesthetic properties, i.e., lidocaine, mixed with epinephrine 1:200,000). The pledgets containing the local anesthetic should be left in place for 5 to 10 minutes. The skin is infiltrated with local anesthetic starting along the base of the nares. This is continued as a subcutaneous infiltration up the nasal facial groove, thereby blocking contributions from the first and second divisions. After topicalization and shrinkage of the nasal mucosa the sphenopalatine ganglion is more easily anesthetized. Dilute local anesthetic with epinephrine 1:200,000 is advised for the external infiltrations.

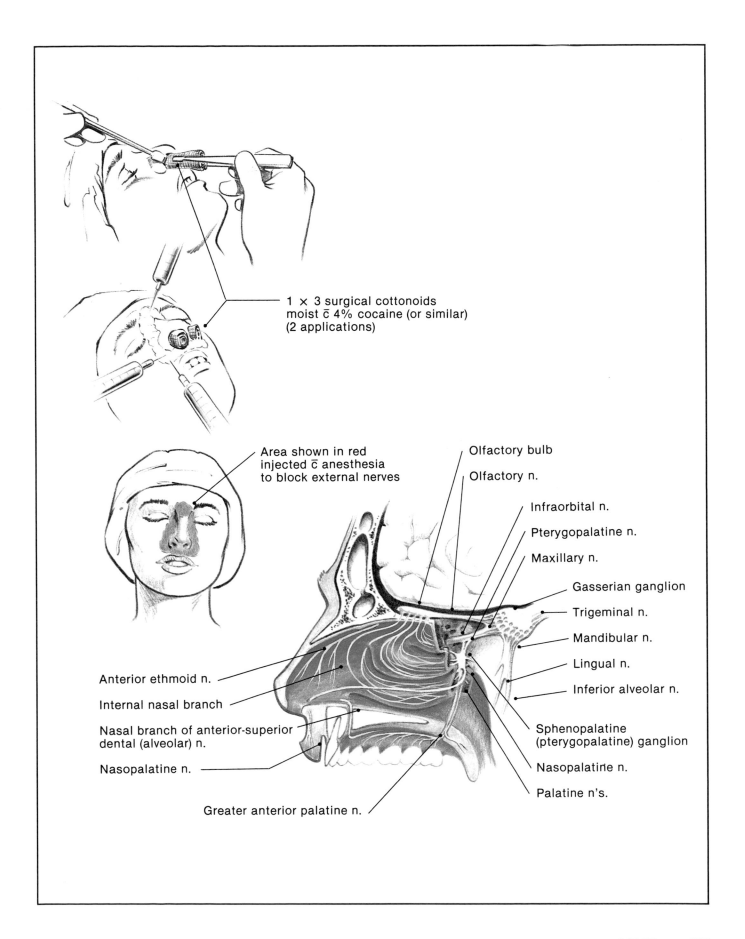

1 × 3 surgical cottonoids
moist c̄ 4% cocaine (or similar)
(2 applications)

Area shown in red
injected c̄ anesthesia
to block external nerves

Olfactory bulb

Olfactory n.

Infraorbital n.

Pterygopalatine n.

Maxillary n.

Gasserian ganglion

Trigeminal n.

Mandibular n.

Lingual n.

Inferior alveolar n.

Sphenopalatine
(pterygopalatine) ganglion

Nasopalatine n.

Palatine n's.

Anterior ethmoid n.

Internal nasal branch

Nasal branch of anterior-superior
dental (alveolar) n.

Nasopalatine n.

Greater anterior palatine n.

Ear

Anatomy

The ear is innervated inferiorly by the greater auricular nerve and anteriorly by branches of the fifth cranial nerve. The ear canal and its lateral surface contain branches of the seventh, ninth, and tenth cranial nerves.

Technique

Infiltration is started inferiorly and advanced close to the substance of the external ear in a posterior direction, thus blocking the major contribution from the greater auricular nerve. The subcutaneous infiltration is continued circumferentially around the ear. This will provide satisfactory anesthesia for the posterior and medial surfaces.

For anesthesia of the anterior lateral surface and external auditory canal, employ a four-quadrant block of the canal using approximately ¼ cc of local anesthetic at 12, 3, 6, and 9 o'clock. The addition of ½ cc of local anesthetic posteriorly into the concha should provide total anesthesia for outer-ear surgery.

Note: If middle-ear surgery is contemplated, the posterior wall of the auditory canal is infiltrated to the tympanic membrane with 1 to 2 cc of local anesthetic.

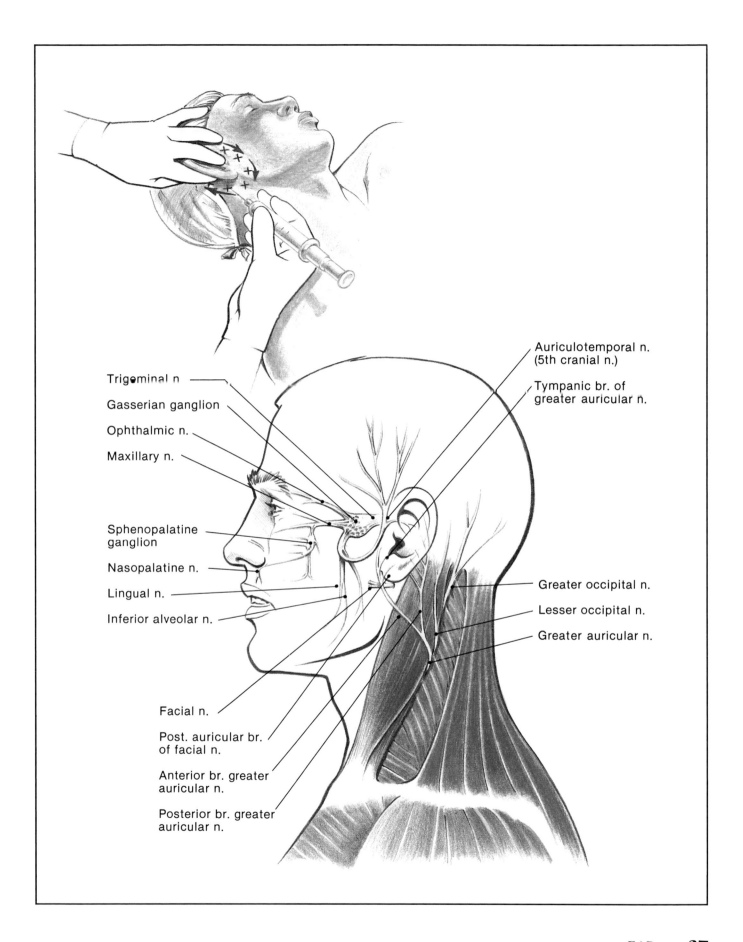

Auriculotemporal n.
(5th cranial n.)

Tympanic br. of
greater auricular n.

Trigeminal n

Gasserian ganglion

Ophthalmic n.

Maxillary n.

Sphenopalatine
ganglion

Nasopalatine n.

Lingual n.

Inferior alveolar n.

Greater occipital n.

Lesser occipital n.

Greater auricular n.

Facial n.

Post. auricular br.
of facial n.

Anterior br. greater
auricular n.

Posterior br. greater
auricular n.

Neck

Cervical Plexus

DEEP BLOCK

Anatomy

The cervical plexus is formed by the ventral primary rami of the first four cervical nerves. Each nerve divides into an ascending and descending branch which communicates with the nerves above and below, respectively. These series of nerve loops form the cervical plexus. The first cervical nerve has no cutaneous distribution, although the others do. The major cutaneous branches of interest are the lesser occipital nerve, the greater auricular nerve, and the suprascapular nerves. Of the muscular branches the most important is the phrenic nerve. Other motor branches supply the muscles of the neck, including the scalenes.

Technique

The patient is positioned supine on the table with face turned away from the side to be blocked. The tip of the mastoid process is identified, as is the insertion of the sternocleidomastoid muscle on the clavicle. The line between these points is usually just anterior to the transverse processes of the cervical vertebrae, the cornu of which are almost always easy to palpate through the skin. Approximately 1 inch below the tip of the mastoid process a skin wheal is made and a 2-inch block needle is inserted. This should be over the cornu of the transverse process of C2. The needle is inserted in a slight caudad direction until the tip of the transverse process is contacted, usually from ½ to 1½ inches, depending on the thickness of the soft tissue. Paresthesias are not sought. Needles should be similarly inserted approximately ½ to 1 inch apart in a caudad direction to block C3 and C4. Three to five cubic centimeters of solution is injected through each needle after careful aspiration for blood and CSF.

Note: The absolute distance from the tip of the mastoid to the cornu of C2 to C4 will vary depending on the length of the neck. All needles should be at approximately the same depth. If there is a disparity in depth, the most superficial needle contacting bone is the correctly positioned one, since needles may inadvertently contact the transverse process proximal to the cornu toward the body of the vertebrae. To obtain a successful block, the needle tip must be at the cornu.

Note: A slight caudad direction of the needle is necessary in order to prevent it from slipping between the transverse processes and possibly injecting local anesthetic into the vertebral artery, epidural space, or subarachnoid space.

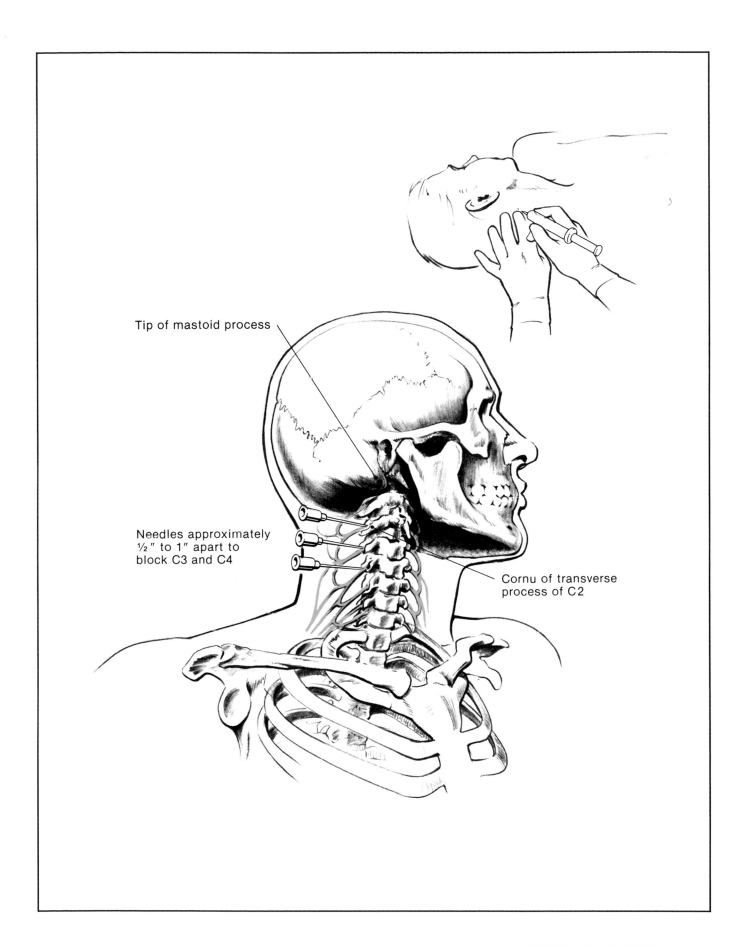

Tip of mastoid process

Needles approximately ½″ to 1″ apart to block C3 and C4

Cornu of transverse process of C2

Superficial Cervical Plexus

Anatomy

The superficial branches of the cervical plexus merge from behind the midpoint of the sternocleidomastoid muscle to supply the overlying skin of the neck from the base of the skull and mandible to the shoulders and clavicle.

Technique

The head is turned away from the side to be blocked. The patient is asked to raise his or her head against mild resistance of the operator's hand. This outlines the sternocleidomastoid muscle quite easily. Along its posterior border and midway between its origin on the clavicle and insertion on the mastoid, a skin wheal is raised. A 2-inch block needle is inserted and 10 cc of solution is infiltrated as the needle is advanced from 1 to 2 inches superiorly and inferiorly along the edge of the muscle. Paresthesias are not sought.

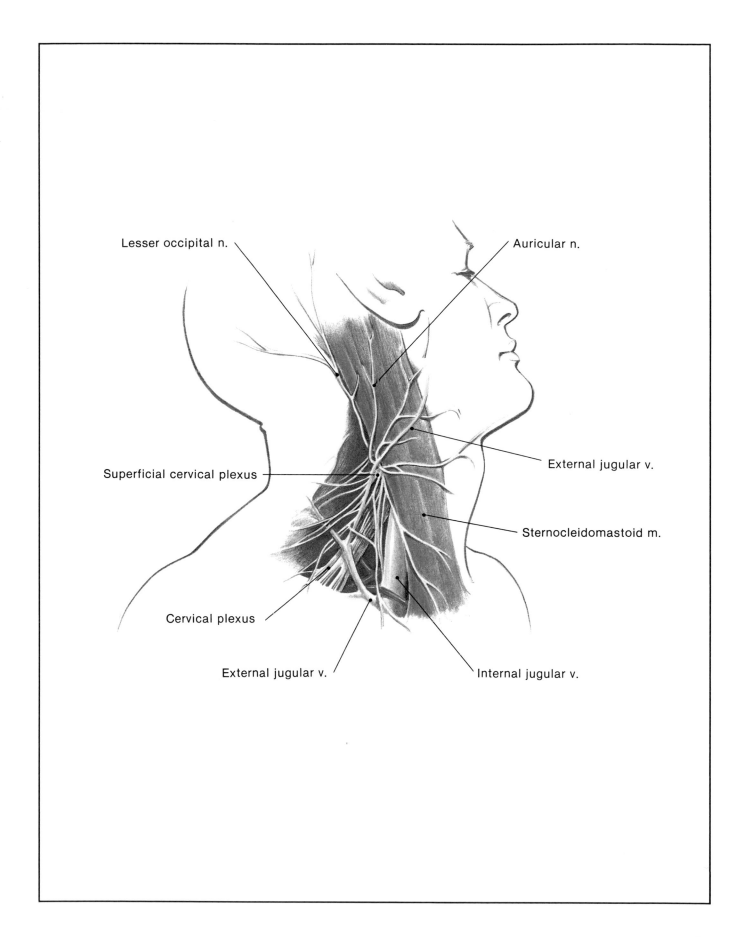

Lesser occipital n.

Auricular n.

External jugular v.

Superficial cervical plexus

Sternocleidomastoid m.

Cervical plexus

External jugular v.

Internal jugular v.

Greater and Lesser Occipital Nerves

Anatomy

The greater occipital nerve arises from the dorsal primary ramus of the second cervical nerve together with a smaller branch of the third cervical nerve. It supplies the medial part of the posterior portion of the scalp.

The lesser occipital nerve arises from the ventral primary rami of the second and third cervical segments. It passes upward along the posterior border of the sternocleidomastoid muscle to supply the cranial surface of the pinna and adjacent scalp.

Technique

This block is done with patient in the sitting position, head slightly flexed so that the chin lies close to the chest. A skin wheal is raised midway between the midline of the neck and the posterior border of the mastoid process at the level of the superior nuchal line. It is usually possible to palpate the occipital artery at this point. A 1-inch needle is inserted perpendicularly until the needle approaches the occipital bone. Paresthesia may be encountered. If not, 5 cc of solution is injected immediately adjacent to the occipital artery in a fanwise distribution, thus blocking the greater occipital nerve.

The lesser occipital nerve and some superficial branches arising from the greater occipital nerve will be blocked by infiltration between the skin and periosteum just below the nuchal ridge. *See also* techniques for Scalp (p. 2) and Superficial Cervical Plexus (p. 42).

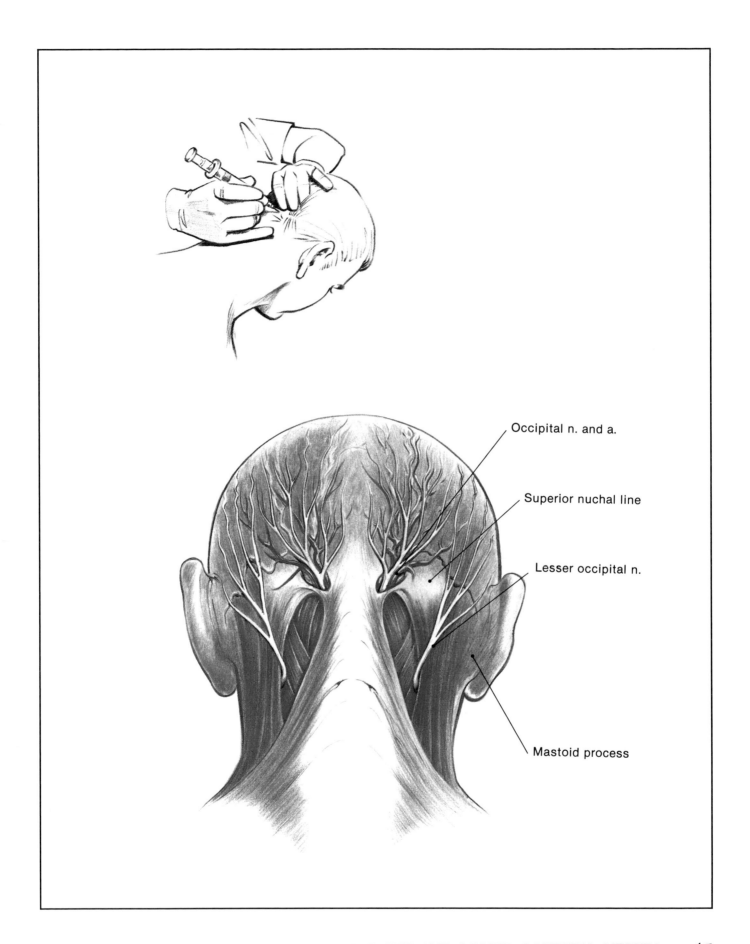

Occipital n. and a.

Superior nuchal line

Lesser occipital n.

Mastoid process

Greater Auricular Nerve

Anatomy

The greater auricular nerve arises from the primary ventral rami of C2 and C3. From there it passes upward and forward, curving around the sternocleidomastoid muscle and becoming superficial to supply the skin in the region of the ear, angle of the jaw, and over the parotid gland.

Technique

This nerve is usually blocked using the same technique as for the superficial cervical plexus (p. 42), of which it is a component.

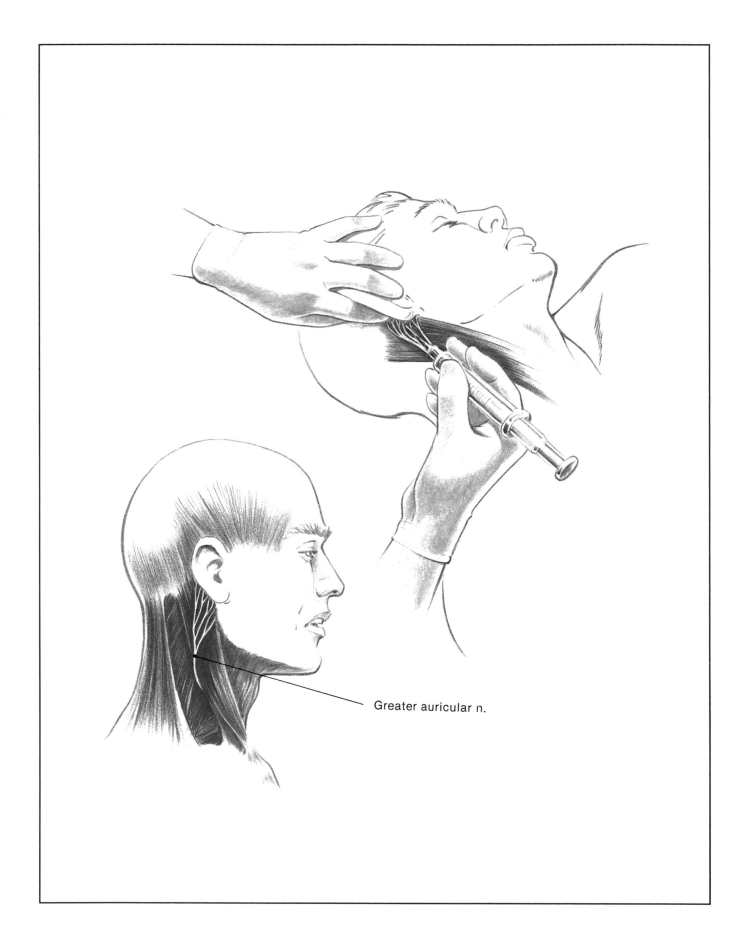

Greater auricular n.

Phrenic Nerve

Anatomy

The phrenic nerves arise from the primary ventral rami of the fourth cervical nerves. They also receive contributions from C3 and C5. The nerves pass downward on the anterior scalene muscles, between them and the omohyoid and sternocleidomastoid muscles. They exit the neck between the subclavian arteries and veins to enter the thorax. The nerves descend through the mediastinal area, over the root of the corresponding-side lung. The right phrenic nerve is closely related in its course to the vena cava. It pierces the diaphragm to supply its right dome on the inferior surface. The left phrenic nerve moves down the thorax adjacent to the left vagus. It then pierces the diaphragm close to the apex of the heart to supply the inferior surface of its left dome.

Technique

The patient lies supine, head turned away from the side to be blocked. Against gentle pressure of the operator's hand, the patient is requested to lift his or her head, thus identifying the lateral border of the sternocleidomastoid muscle. Just lateral to the sternocleidomastoid, between it and the anterior scalene muscle at about an inch above the clavicle, a skin wheal is raised. A 3-inch, 22-gauge block needle is inserted parallel to the scalene muscle in the groove between the scalene muscle and the sternocleidomastoid. At about 1 inch in depth, 8 to 10 cc of local anesthetic is infiltrated as the needle is moved slowly back and forth for a short distance medially and laterally. No paresthesias are sought.

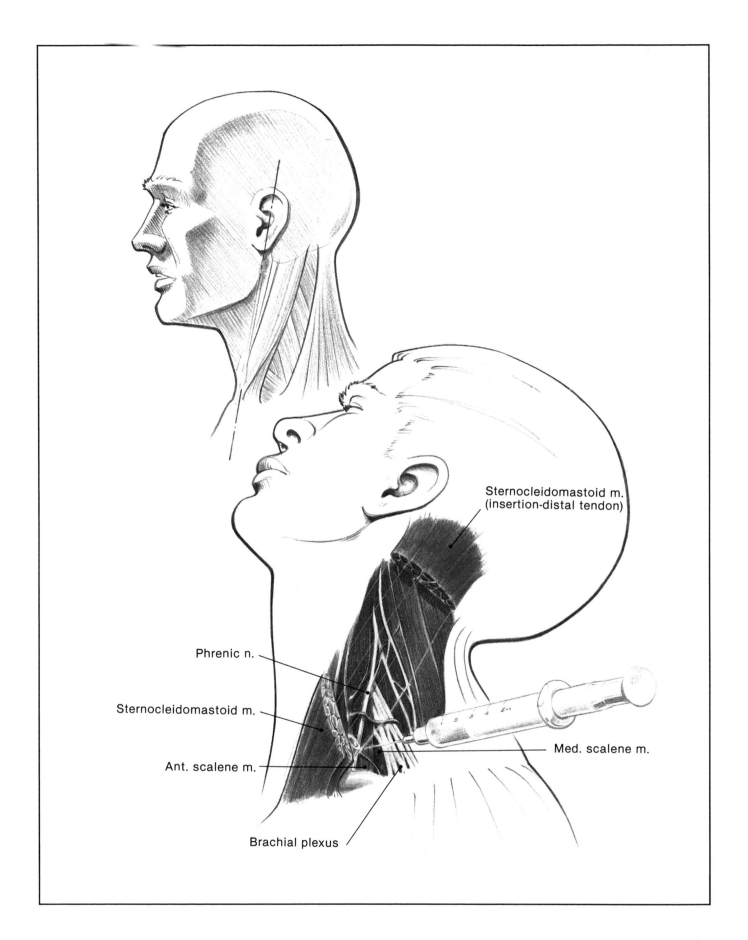

Sternocleidomastoid m.
(insertion-distal tendon)

Phrenic n.

Sternocleidomastoid m.

Ant. scalene m.

Med. scalene m.

Brachial plexus

Stellate Ganglion

Anatomy

The stellate ganglion is in most cases the fusion of the inferior cervical and first thoracic sympathetic ganglia. It is usually an oval-shaped mass approximately 1 inch long and ½ inch wide located in front of the head of the first rib and the transverse process of the seventh cervical vertebrae. It lies deep to the subclavian artery, approximately at the origin of the vertebral artery. Surrounding the ganglion are (1) the bony structures mentioned above posteriorly, (2) the dome of the pleura inferiorly, (3) the scalene muscle mass laterally, (4) the vertebral column medially, and (5) the contents of the carotid sheath anteriorly. It should also be noted that the longus colli muscle, which lies over the transverse processes of the cervical vertebrae, separates the ganglion from the bony transverse process itself.

Technique

The patient lies supine. A small pillow or folded towel is placed underneath the shoulders and the head is extended and kept midline. The medial (sternal) head of the clavicle is palpated, as is the trachea. One and a half to two inches above the clavicle, just parallel to the lateral edge of the trachea on the involved side, the contents of the carotid sheath are drawn laterally by the palpating fingers. A 1½- to 3-inch needle is inserted perpendicular and just lateral to the trachea, between the trachea and the retracted carotid sheath. The needle is advanced until the transverse process of C6 or C7 is encountered, then withdrawn 1 to 2 mm to remove the needle tip from the longus colli muscle. After careful aspiration, 8 to 10 cc of the local anesthetic solution is injected.

In the average patient the needle should strike the transverse process at a depth of approximately 1 inch. In heavier and thicker necks it may go as deep as 1½ to 2 inches. If the needle goes further than this, it has entered the space between the transverse processes. It should be withdrawn and redirected in a slightly cephalad direction.

If a block of the sympathetic supply to the arm is required, the patient should be raised to about a 30 degree sitting position after the local anesthetic is injected and the needle removed. This allows the local anesthetic to diffuse down to the upper thoracic sympathetic ganglia.

Note: Careful aspiration must be part of the blocking technique, since the needle is extremely close to the vertebral artery. Even a small amount of local anesthetic, a drop or two, into the vertebral artery may cause convulsions. If the needle is directed too caudad it is possible to puncture the dome of the pleura. Since the results of the block are similar when either the C7 or C6 transverse process is contacted, it is best to place the needle slightly higher in the neck.

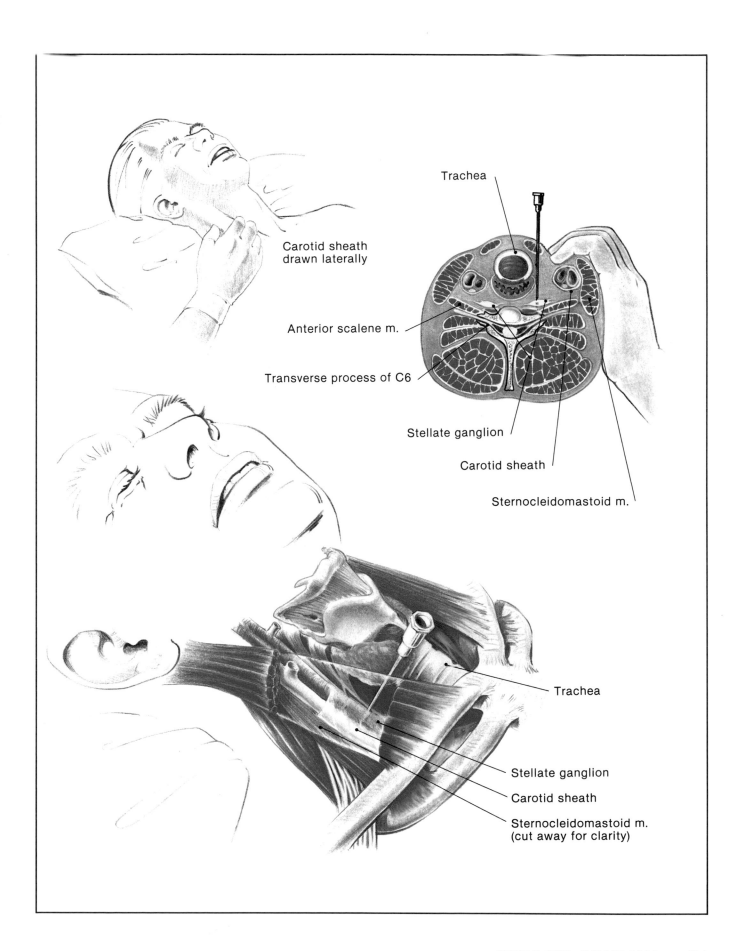

Trachea

Carotid sheath
drawn laterally

Anterior scalene m.

Transverse process of C6

Stellate ganglion

Carotid sheath

Sternocleidomastoid m.

Trachea

Stellate ganglion

Carotid sheath

Sternocleidomastoid m.
(cut away for clarity)

Glossopharyngeal and Vagus Nerves

Anatomy

The glossopharyngeal nerve originates as a series of rootlets from a groove in the medulla between the olive and the inferior cerebellar peduncle. The rootlets fuse to form a single nerve that exits the skull via the jugular foramen and passes anteriorly between the internal jugular vein and internal carotid artery, going medial to the styloid process and lateral to the vagus and spinal accessory nerves. The terminal branches of the nerve include (1) the tympanic nerve to the middle ear, (2) the carotid nerve to the baroreceptors of the carotid sinus and chemoreceptors of the carotid body, (3) the pharyngeal nerve, which is mainly sensory to the pharyngeal mucosa, (4) tonsillar nerves to the mucosa over the palatine tonsil and adjacent parts of the soft palate, and (5) sensory branches to the posterior one-third of the tongue.

The vagus nerve also originates from the groove between the olive and the inferior cerebellar peduncle. Its fibers are slightly caudad to the fibers that make up the glossopharyngeal nerve. It exits the skull via the jugular foramen in close contact with the spinal accessory nerve. After leaving the skull, the vagus nerve lies in the carotid sheath between the internal jugular vein and the internal carotid artery.

Major vagus nerve branches in the head and neck are (1) the meningeal to the dura mater of the posterior cranial fossa; (2) the auricular to the posterior wall of the external auditory meatus and lower part of the tympanic membrane; (3) the pharyngeal, major motor supply of the pharyngeal muscle; (4) the superior laryngeal, which supplies the mucous membranes of the pharynx and larynx from the posterior part of the dorsum of the tongue to the vocal cords; and (5) the recurrent laryngeal, which supplies the intrinsic muscles of the larynx and the mucous membranes of the pharynx and larynx below the vocal cords. There are also cardiac, thoracic, bronchial, and vascular branches in the thorax, as well as multiple abdominal branches.

Technique

The patient lies supine, head in the neutral position. The anterior border of the mastoid process is identified. A skin wheal is made immediately below the external auditory meatus and just anterior to the anterior border of the mastoid process. A 2-inch needle is inserted perpendicular to the skin. At a depth of from ½ to 1 inch, the styloid process should be contacted. The needle is then redirected to go just posterior to the styloid process and advanced an additional ½ to 1 inch. At this point the needle tip should be opposite the opening of the jugular foramen. After careful aspiration, 3 to 5 cc of local anesthetic is injected.

Note: The spinal accessory and hypoglossal nerves are usually blocked when the above technique is used.

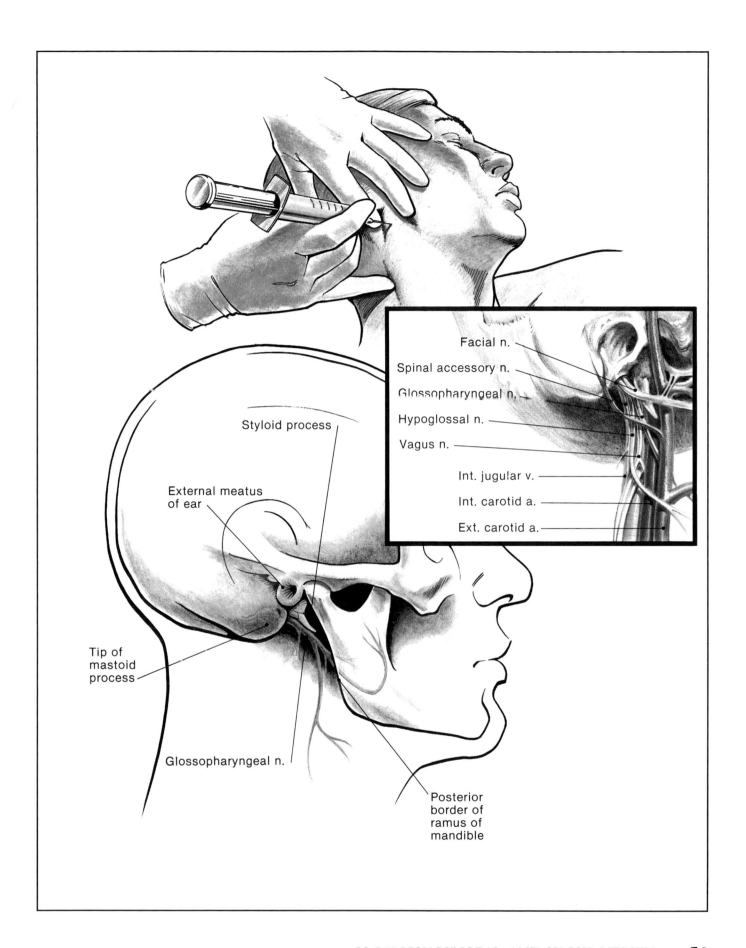

Facial n.

Spinal accessory n.

Glossopharyngeal n.

Hypoglossal n.

Vagus n.

Int. jugular v.

Int. carotid a.

Ext. carotid a.

Styloid process

External meatus
of ear

Tip of
mastoid
process

Glossopharyngeal n.

Posterior
border of
ramus of
mandible

Spinal Accessory (11th Cranial) Nerve

Anatomy

The spinal accessory nerve has two roots—cranial and spinal. The cranial root arises from the nucleus ambiguus and is attached to the medulla in the retroolivary sulcus by a series of rootlets. The cranial root joins the vagus nerve to be distributed to the muscles of the pharynx and larynx.

The spinal root originates from the spinal nucleus, a column of motor neurons that exists in the upper six cervical segments of the spinal cord. These fibers pass cranially and unite to form a single bundle that enters the skull via the foramen magnum. Combined cranial and spinal roots then leave the skull through the jugular foramen in the same dural sheath as the vagal trunk. Spinal fibers pass downward and backward as a single nerve trunk that enters and supplies the upper part of the sternocleidomastoid muscle, eventually emerging from its posterior border somewhere in the upper third of the muscle. In combination with branches of the cervical plexus it innervates the trapezius muscle.

Technique

The spinal accessory nerve emerges from underneath the sternocleidomastoid muscle at approximately the junction of the upper and middle thirds posteriorly. Block is best accomplished here. The area adjacent to the sternocleidomastoid muscle is infiltrated in a fan-wise distribution with about 10 cc of local anesthetic.

Note: Many times this nerve is blocked while doing a superficial cervical plexus block and vice versa.

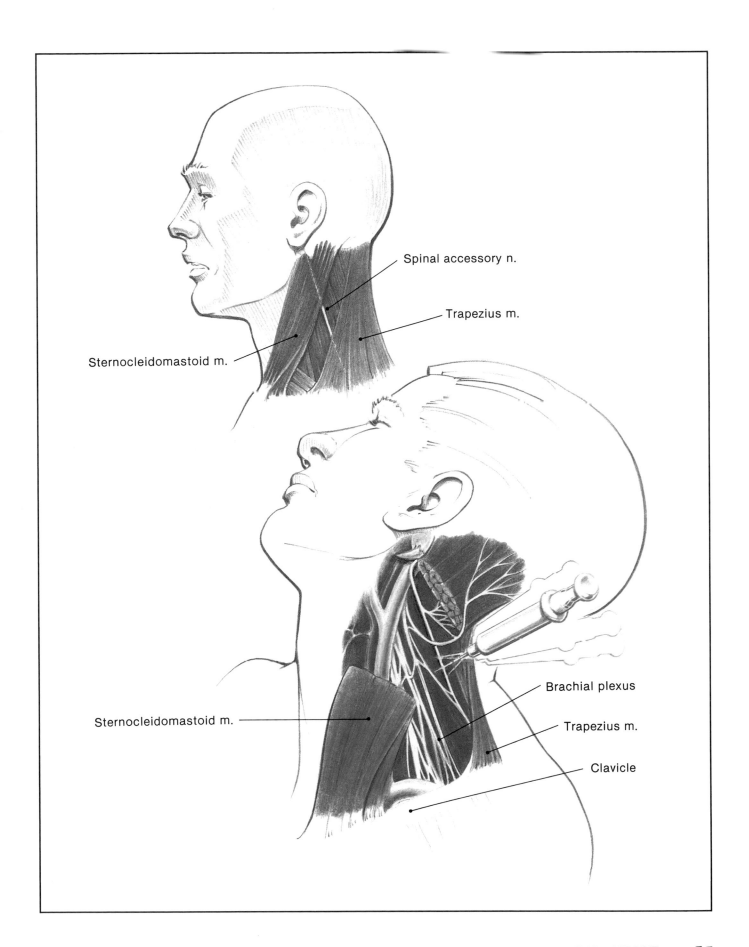

Spinal accessory n.

Trapezius m.

Sternocleidomastoid m.

Sternocleidomastoid m.

Brachial plexus

Trapezius m.

Clavicle

SPINAL ACCESSORY (11TH CRANIAL) NERVE **55**

Larynx

Anatomy

Nerve supply to the mucous membranes of the larynx is from the superior and recurrent laryngeal nerves. The superior laryngeal nerve is primarily vagal in origin, with a small branch also coming from the superior cervical ganglion. It descends laterally to the pharynx, behind the internal carotid artery, and at the level of the hyoid divides into internal and external branches. The internal branch in turn also divides into superior and inferior twigs. The superior component is sensory to the mucous membranes of the lower part of the pharynx, epiglottis, vallecula, and vestibule of the larynx. The inferior nerve provides sensation to the aryepiglottic folds and mucous membranes above the level of the cords.

The mucous membranes below the level of the vocal cords is supplied by branches from the recurrent laryngeal nerve. All intrinsic muscles of the larynx are supplied by the recurrent laryngeal nerve except the cricothyroid muscle, which is innervated by the external laryngeal nerve.

Technique

For Transtrachial Nerve Block. The patient lies supine, the head slightly extended. The inferior portion of the thyroid cartilage and the cricoid cartilages are identified. Between these cartilages the thumb and forefinger stabilize the trachea. A 1-inch, 22-gauge needle is securely fastened to a syringe and inserted through the cricothyroid ligament into the trachea. After gentle aspiration that should produce air, 3 to 4 cc of a concentrated local anesthetic is injected.

Note: Since the patient will cough vigorously when the local anesthetic is injected, the procedure should be done extremely rapidly and the needle withdrawn as soon as possible.

See p. 58 for block of the superior laryngeal nerve.

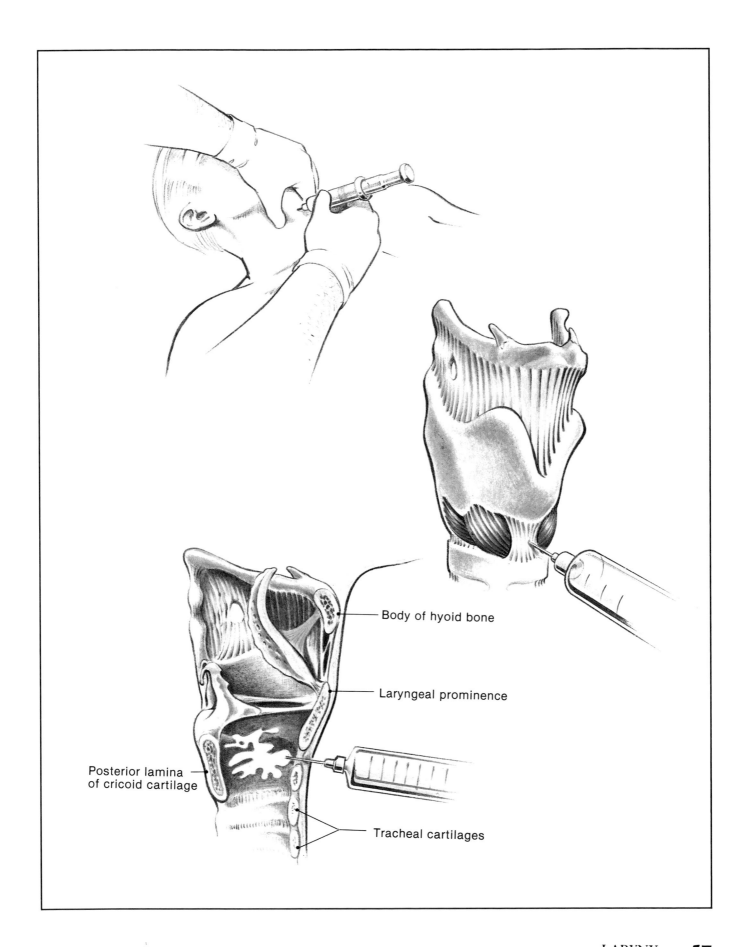

Body of hyoid bone

Laryngeal prominence

Posterior lamina
of cricoid cartilage

Tracheal cartilages

Superior Laryngeal Nerve

Anatomy

The superior laryngeal nerve, a branch of the vagus nerve, passes downward and forward deep to the internal and external carotid arteries toward the thyroid cartilage. The internal laryngeal nerve, largest sensory branch, pierces the thyroid membrane, providing sensation to the mucous membranes of the pharynx and larynx immediately above the glottis. The external laryngeal nerve supplies the cricothyroid muscle. For further details see anatomy of larynx (p. 56).

Technique

With patient in the supine position, head slightly extended, the thyroid cornu and cornu of the hyoid cartilage are palpated in the lateral aspect of the neck. At a point between these, perpendicular to the skin, a ½-inch, 25-gauge block needle is inserted. A slight popping sensation may be felt when the needle pierces the thyrohyoid ligament. Two cubic centimeters of local anesthetic is injected. Paresthesias are not sought.

Note: In the very heavy neck a 1-inch needle might be required.

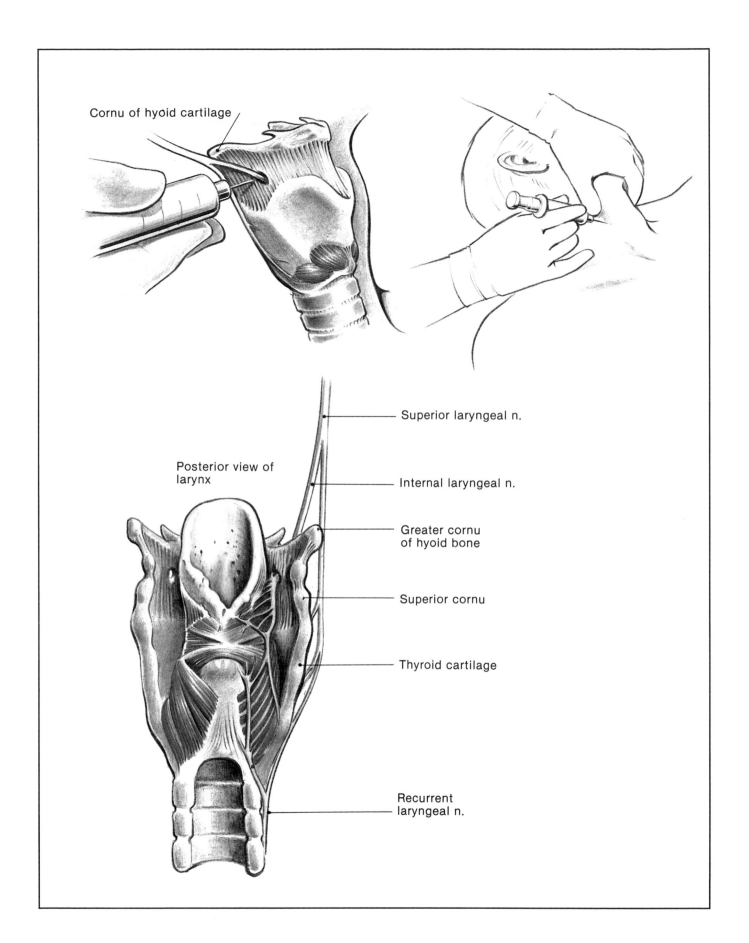

Cornu of hyoid cartilage

Posterior view of larynx

Superior laryngeal n.

Internal laryngeal n.

Greater cornu of hyoid bone

Superior cornu

Thyroid cartilage

Recurrent laryngeal n.

Recurrent Laryngeal Nerves

Anatomy

The recurrent laryngeal nerves, branches of the vagus, have differing anatomy on the right and left sides. On the right side, after the vagus crosses in front of the subclavian artery, the right recurrent laryngeal loops below the subclavian artery and ascends behind the carotid sheath between the trachea and the esophagus. The left nerve arises from the left vagus as it crosses the aortic arch looping below the ligamentum arteriosum ascending behind the aorta to reach the groove between the esophagus and trachea. At the level of the cricoid cartilage both nerves pass beneath the lower border of the inferior constrictor muscle to enter the larynx. The recurrent laryngeal nerve supplies all of the intrinsic muscles of the larynx, with the exception of the cricothyroid muscle. It is the sensory supply to the mucous membranes of the trachea below the level of the vocal cords.

Technique

Although the nerves can be blocked individually in the groove between the esophagus and trachea, the terminal sensory branches are anesthetized using the transtracheal approach (*see* p. 56).

Upper Extremity

Brachial Plexus

INTERSCALENE APPROACH

Anatomy

The brachial plexus is formed in the neck from the ventral primary rami of the fifth, sixth, seventh, and eighth cervical nerves and the first thoracic nerve. C4 and T2 may also contribute fibers to the plexus. The roots, as just described, course between the anterior scalene and middle scalene muscles on their way to the arm.

At the lateral border of the middle scalene muscle, rami from the fifth, sixth, and perhaps fourth cervical nerves unite to form a single bundle called the upper trunk. The primary ramus from the seventh nerve continues as the middle trunk and the primary rami of the eighth cervical, first thoracic, and sometimes second thoracic nerves form the lower trunk. The trunks proceed laterally and inferiorly to leave the neck and enter the axilla between the clavicle and first rib.

At this point the trunks of the plexus divide into anterior and posterior divisions. Anterior divisions of the upper and middle trunks, which contain fibers from the fifth, sixth, seventh, and sometimes fourth cervical nerves unite to form the lateral cord of the brachial plexus. The anterior division of the lower trunk contains fibers from the eighth cervical nerve and the first and perhaps second thoracic roots and continues as the medial cord. The dorsal divisions of all the cervical nerves, and to a lesser extent the first thoracic nerve, become the posterior cord.

High in the axilla, at about the level of the lateral border of the pectoralis minor, cords divide into the peripheral nerves of the upper extremity. From the roots of the brachial plexus emanate several nerves going to the scalene and other muscles of the neck, a branch from C5 to the phrenic nerve, and fibers from C5, C6, and C7 to the long thoracic nerve. The upper trunk also provides a nerve to the subclavian muscle as well as the suprascapular nerve from its C4, C5, and C6 components.

The important peripheral branches of the lateral cord are the musculocutaneous nerve and the lateral root of the median nerve, both originating from C5, C6, and C7. From the medial cord (C8 and T1) comes the medial root of the median nerve, the ulnar nerve, and the medial cutaneous nerves of the arm and forearm.

The posterior cord gives rise to the subscapular nerves, the axillary nerve, and the radial nerve, which gets its components from C5 through T1.

The scalene muscles are encapsulated by an extension of the prevertebral fascia. This effectively limits dispersion of local anesthetics. The fascia continues to surround the neurovascular complex as it proceeds from between the scalene muscles into the upper arm.

Technique

The patient lies supine, head turned away from the side to be blocked and chin tilted slightly upward. The shoulder on the ipsilateral side is depressed by having the patient reach for the knee. The lateral edge of the clavicular insertion of the sternocleidomastoid muscle is identified by having the patient lift the head against gentle resistance. At the C6 level (approximately) the operator's fingers roll over the lateral edge of the sternocleidomastoid muscle and onto the belly of the anterior scalene muscle. The fingers are then moved laterally, thus identifying the groove between the anterior scalene and middle scalene muscles, which in most patients is a subtle depression. A skin wheal is raised and 1 ½-inch, 23-gauge blunt tip block needle is inserted parallel to the bellies of the scalene muscles and into the groove between them. The needle should be at right angles to the skin of the neck and thus slightly caudad in direction as it advances. Paresthesias from the upper components of the brachial plexus, usually to the shoulder or upper arm, should be elicited when the needle is from ½ to 1 inch deep, depending on the size of the neck. Once a definite paresthesia from any root of the plexus is obtained, 30 to 40 cc of local anesthetic is injected. The area immediately above the site of injection, at the level of the C4 or C5 transverse process, is compressed, allowing the local anesthetic solution to bathe the brachial plexus rather than diffuse in a cephalad direction.

Note: Paresthesias are required to locate the plexus with certainty.

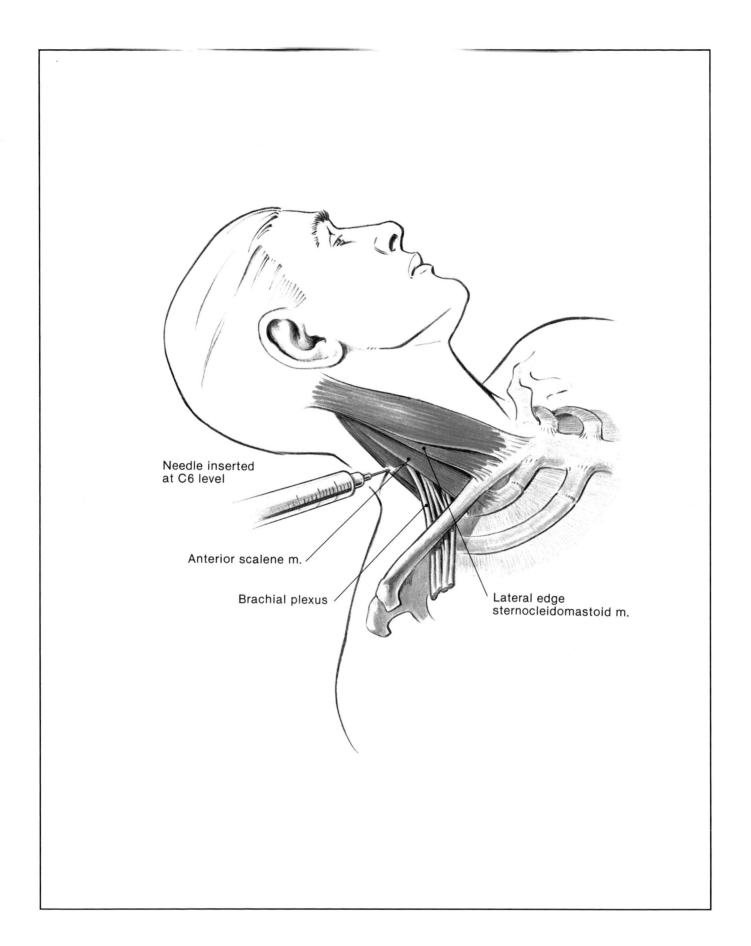

Needle inserted
at C6 level

Anterior scalene m.

Brachial plexus

Lateral edge
sternocleidomastoid m.

Brachial Plexus

SUPRACLAVICULAR APPROACH

Anatomy

See anatomy for Brachial Plexus—Interscalene Approach (p. 62).

Technique

The patient is positioned as for the interscalene approach and again the groove between the scalene muscles is identified. Palpation of the subclavian artery is attempted. The subclavian artery lies between the scalene muscles, just behind the clavicle. A 1½- to 2-inch, 23-gauge needle is inserted at the C5 to C6 level between the scalene muscles, directed caudally toward the subclavian artery and first rib, and advanced slowly. A paresthesia is usually elicited almost immediately after the needle has entered the interscalene groove. If not, the needle is further advanced toward the artery and first rib. If a depth of 1 ½ inch has been reached with no paresthesias elicited, the artery not entered, or the rib not met, the landmarks should be rechecked and the procedure repeated. Once a paresthesia is noted, 25 to 30 cc of local anesthetic is injected.

Note: It is not wise to proceed with longer needles since the first rib may be bypassed and the pleural cavity entered. If the artery is entered prior to a paresthesia occurring, the needle should be withdrawn from the artery and the local anesthetic injected after confirming that the needle tip is extravascular by frequent aspirations.

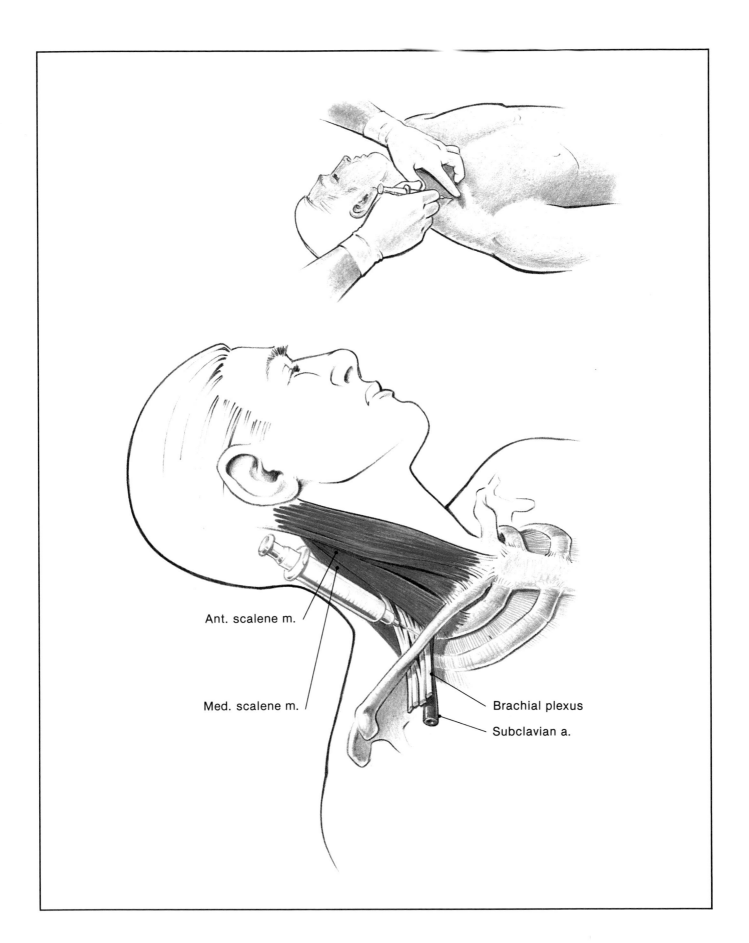

Ant. scalene m.

Med. scalene m.

Brachial plexus

Subclavian a.

Brachial Plexus

INFRACLAVICULAR APPROACH

Anatomy

See anatomy for Brachial Plexus—Interscalene Approach (p. 62).

Technique

The patient lies supine, shoulder and arm in the neutral position. The middle of the clavicle is identified and a skin wheal is raised 1 inch inferior to it. A 3-inch block needle is advanced laterally in the general direction of the head of the humerus. The subclavian artery should be palpated as far laterally as possible. This adds another landmark to which the needle should be directed. As the needle passes deep to the clavicle and toward the artery, a paresthesia of one of the branches of the brachial plexus should be encountered at a depth of from 2 to 2½ inches. Since a paresthesia is required for successful block, the needle tip should be repositioned until one is obtained. Once an adequate paresthesia is achieved, 20 to 30 cc of local anesthetic is deposited after careful aspiration. Aspiration should be repeated several times during the injection to make sure the needle tip has not entered any major vessel.

Note: The general direction of the needle is away from the chest wall, minimizing the risk of pneumothorax.

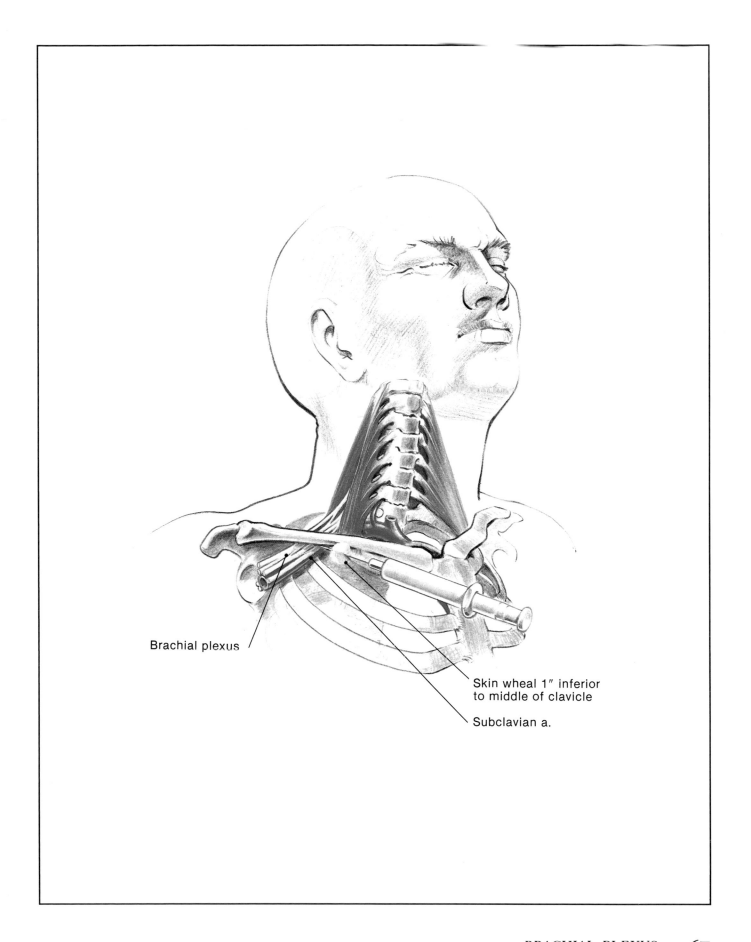

Brachial plexus

Skin wheal 1″ inferior
to middle of clavicle

Subclavian a.

Brachial Plexus

AXILLARY APPROACH

Anatomy

See anatomy of Brachial Plexus—Interscalene Approach (p. 62).

The continuation of the prevertebral fascia in the axilla is known as the axillary sheath, which surrounds the neurovascular complex.

Technique

The patient lies supine, arm abducted to slightly greater than 90 degrees. The axillary artery is palpated as high up in the axilla as possible. Once located, the artery (and therefore the sheath) is digitally compressed. A ¾- to 1½-inch, 23-gauge block needle is inserted just proximal to the point of compression, angling centrally toward the artery. The needle is slowly advanced until the neurovascular compartment is entered by piercing its containing sheath. Paresthesia involving either the median or ulnar nerves is usually obtained. This paresthesia must be a definite one, radiating to the wrist or fingers. Once it has occurred, 30 to 40 cc of local anesthetic is injected into the sheath. During the injection aspiration is performed several times to assure that the needle tip has not inadvertently advanced into the vasculature. Upon completion of the injection digital pressure is maintained on the axillary artery and the arm is brought down to the side. Digital pressure is continued for two minutes. Anesthesia should start within several minutes after injection, with the time to surgical anesthesia varying according to the local anesthetic used.

If paresthesias are impossible to elicit, the following alternate technique may be used. The arm is positioned as above. The axillary artery is approached and entered at a right angle immediately above the palpating finger. The needle is advanced through the artery, piercing its posterior wall. Aspiration should reveal no additional return of blood. Fifteen to twenty cubic centimeters of local anesthetic is deposited deep to the artery, with frequent aspirations assuring that the needle tip remains extravascular. The needle is then withdrawn through the artery. When aspiration for blood is negative, the needle has reentered the sheath superficial to the artery itself. With frequent aspirations an additional 15 to 20 cc of local anesthetic is injected.

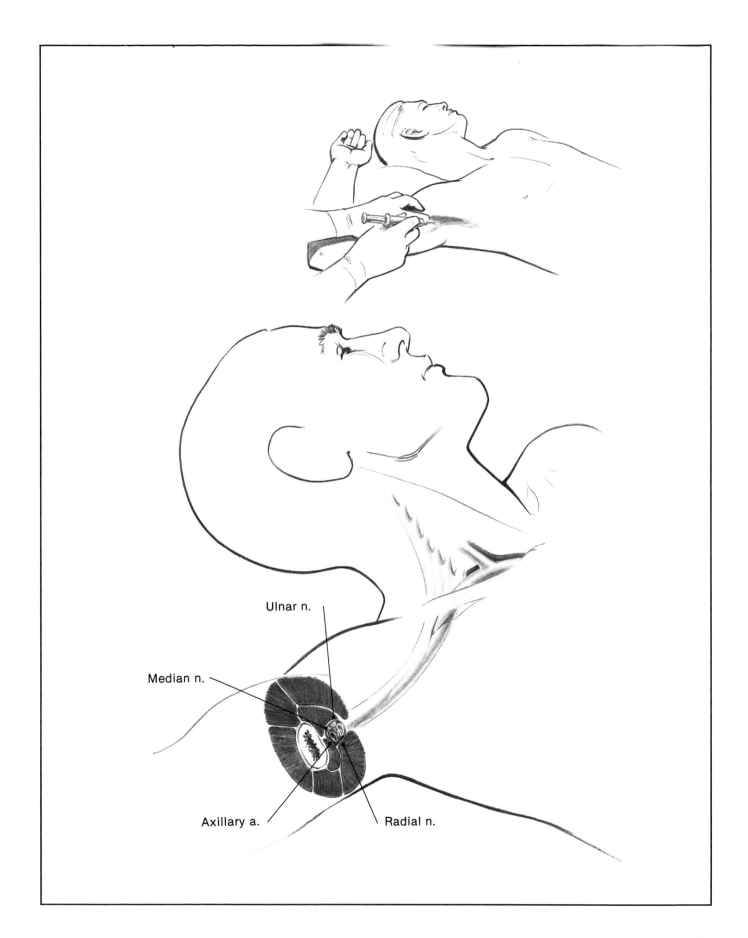

Ulnar n.

Median n.

Axillary a.

Radial n.

Musculocutaneous Nerve

Anatomy

The musculocutaneous nerve originates from the C5, C6, and C7 nerve roots as a branch from the lateral cord. The nerve pierces the coracobrachialis muscle. It then runs between the biceps and the brachialis, sending branches to both of these muscles. After piercing the fascia it continues as the lateral cutaneous nerve providing sensation to radial and posterior skin of the lower half to third of the forearm.

Technique

There are two techniques that can be used to block the musculocutaneous nerve.

Technique 1: Block of the musculocutaneous nerve may be performed at the time of axillary block by redirecting a 1- to 1½-inch, 22-gauge needle just above the axillary sheath (as ordinarily positioned for an axillary block) into the substance of the coracobrachialis muscle and infiltrating 5 to 8 cc of local anesthetic. Paresthesias are not sought.

Technique 2: The sensory continuation of the musculocutaneous nerve—the lateral cutaneous nerve of the forearm—is blocked by inserting a 1- to 1½-inch, 23-gauge block needle just lateral to the tendon of the biceps muscle on a line between the two epicondyles of the humerus. Three cubic centimeters of local anesthetic is injected just deep to the subcutaneous tissue in a fanwise distribution as the needle approaches the bone. An additional subcutaneous infiltration of 1 to 2 cc between the lateral border of the tendon and the radial side of the arm will insure that the few remaining superficial sensory branches of the musculocutaneous nerve are blocked.

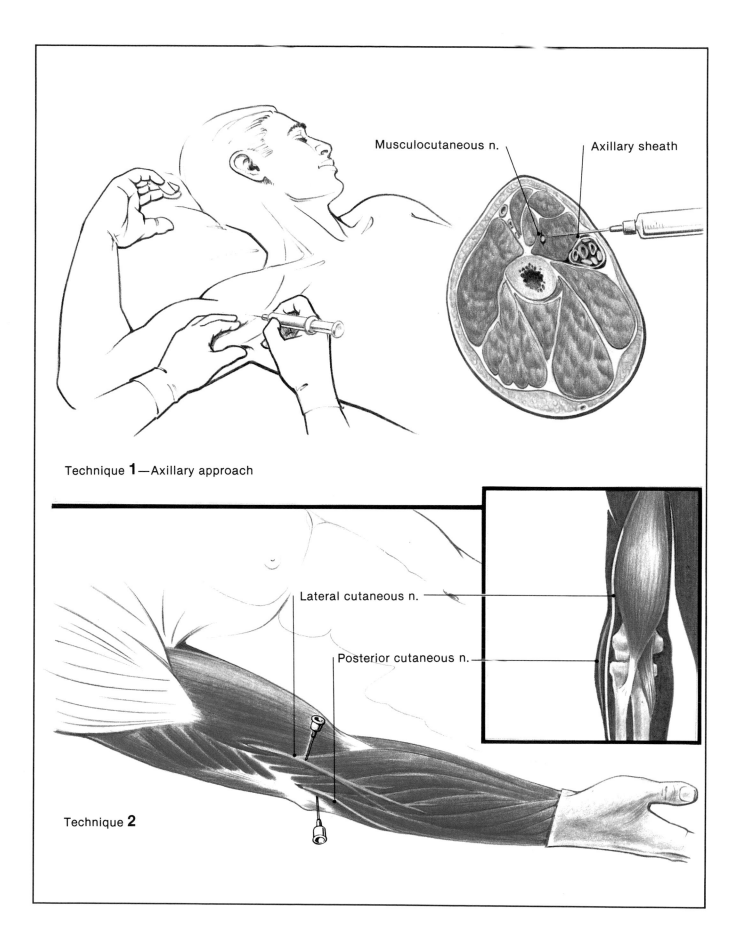

Musculocutaneous n.

Axillary sheath

Technique **1**—Axillary approach

Lateral cutaneous n.

Posterior cutaneous n.

Technique **2**

Suprascapular Nerve

Anatomy

The suprascapular nerve originates from the C5 and C6 nerve roots of the upper trunk of the brachial plexus. A contribution from C4 is usually present as well. The suprascapular nerve descends posteriorly, passing through the scapular notch and innervating the supraspinatus muscle and, more distally, the infraspinatus muscle. It also gives off sensory branches to the shoulder joint.

Technique

This block is done with the patient sitting, head allowed to flex forward. The spine of the scapula is palpated along its entire length, from the medial border of the scapula to the acromial process. At a point 1 inch above the junction of the middle and outer third of the spine a skin wheal is raised. A 3-inch block needle is advanced toward the scapula following the angle the spine makes with the body of the scapula. The body of the scapula should be reached at a depth of about 2 inches. The needle is then moved fanlike from medial to lateral in a plane slightly superior to where the needle first encountered the body of the scapula. The needle tip will lose contact with the bone and enter the suprascapular notch. Eight to ten cubic centimeters of solution should be injected; no paresthesia is sought.

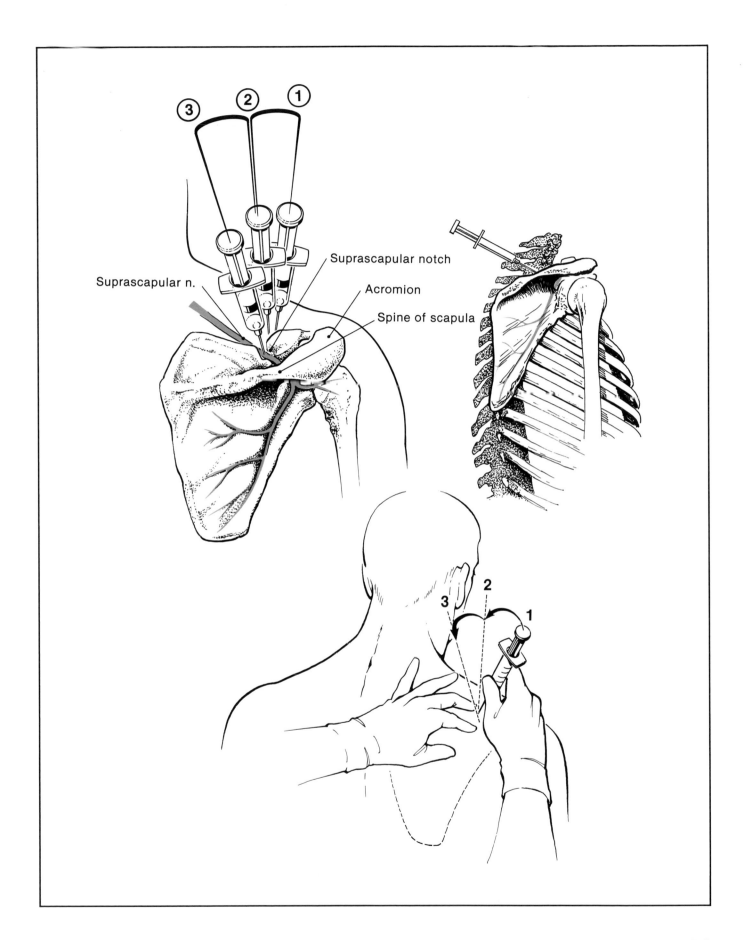

Suprascapular n.

Suprascapular notch

Acromion

Spine of scapula

Intercostobrachial and Medial Cutaneous Nerve of the Arm

Anatomy

The intercostobrachial nerve is the lateral cutaneous branch of the second intercostal nerve. The medial cutaneous nerve originates from the medial cord of the brachial plexus (C8 and T1). Its fibers communicate with those of the intercostobrachial nerve to supply the skin of the axilla and the proximal part of the medial surface of the arm.

Technique

The arm is positioned as for axillary approach to the brachial plexus (p. 68). A subcutaneous infiltration is made to put an arc of local anesthetic superficial to the sheath. From 5 to 8 cc of local anesthetic is used, raising a skin wheal from the biceps to the triceps along the axillary surface of the arm.

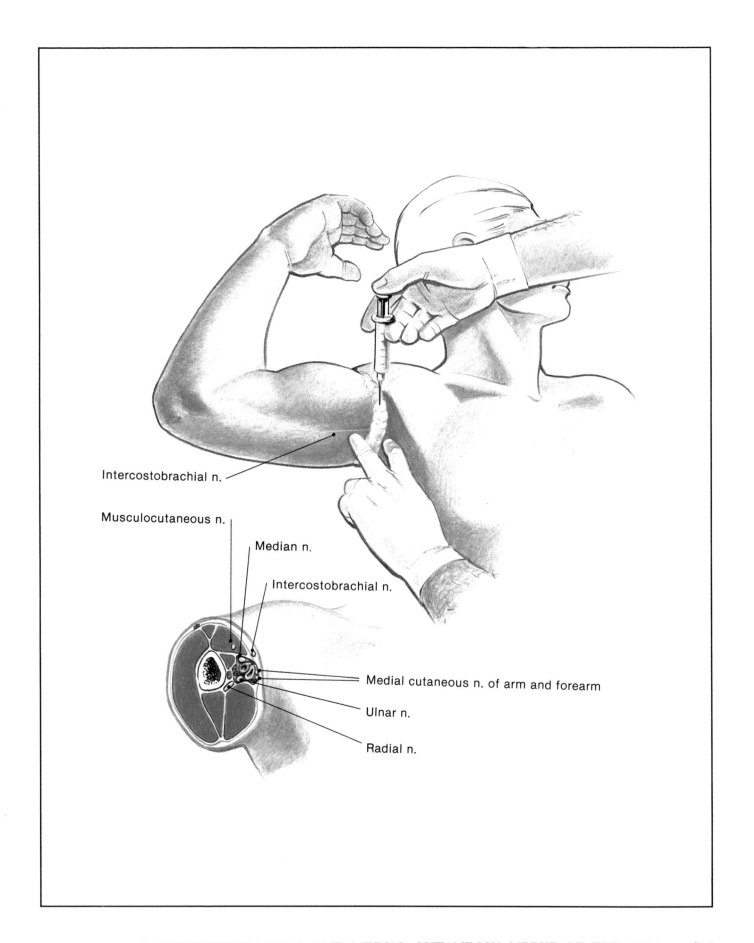

Intercostobrachial n.

Musculocutaneous n.

Median n.

Intercostobrachial n.

Medial cutaneous n. of arm and forearm

Ulnar n.

Radial n.

Radial Nerve

BLOCK IN THE UPPER ARM

Anatomy

The radial nerve arises from the posterior cord and contains fibers from C5 through T1. In the upper arm the nerve lies just posterior to the axillary artery as the major continuation of the posterior cord. After leaving the axilla it inclines backward between the long and medial heads of the triceps muscle running obliquely across the posterior surface of the humerus in the musculospiral groove. It supplies motor branches to the medial long head of the triceps. Just before entering the groove it gives off the posterior cutaneous nerve of the arm; the lateral cutaneous nerve of the arm and posterior cutaneous nerve of the forearm originate a little further down in the groove.

Between the groove and the lateral epicondyle of the humerus, where the radial nerve divides into its two terminal branches, multiple motor fibers are given off. The superficial branch is the direct continuation of the nerve. It descends in the forearm with the radial artery, dividing in the lower forearm into branches that supply the skin of the dorsum of the wrist and dorsal aspects of the lateral 3½ digits. The deep branch, which also originates at the level of the epicondyle, is primarily motor to the extensor muscles of the forearm.

Technique

The arm is extended and the lateral epicondyle of the humerus identified. Three to four inches proximal to this along the lateral aspect of the humerus the radial nerve can often be palpated as it approaches the elbow through the musculospiral groove between the heads of the triceps muscle. Many times the palpating finger can elicit a paresthesia to the back of the hand. A 1-inch, 22-gauge block needle (the size may have to be increased for a very muscular arm) is advanced perpendicular to the lateral aspect of the humerus and the bone contacted. By moving the needle tip in a fanwise motion up and down the bone the nerve will be encountered and paresthesias elicited. Five to eight cubic centimeters of solution is then injected.

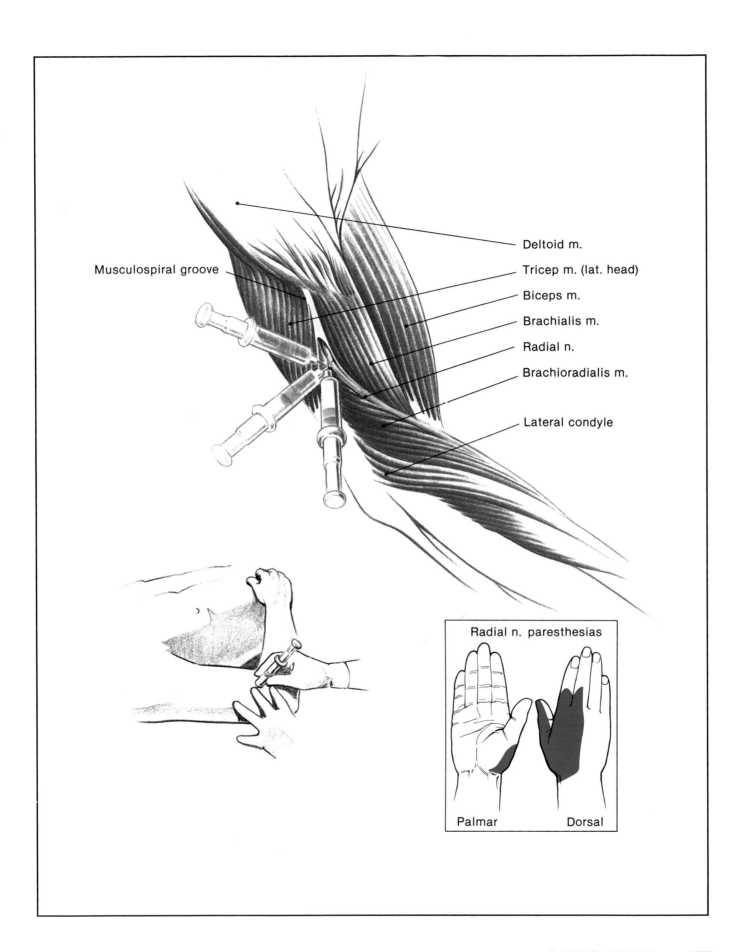

Deltoid m.

Musculospiral groove

Tricep m. (lat. head)

Biceps m.

Brachialis m.

Radial n.

Brachioradialis m.

Lateral condyle

Radial n. paresthesias

Palmar

Dorsal

Radial Nerve

BLOCK AT THE ELBOW

Anatomy

See anatomy for Radial Nerve—Block in the Upper Arm (p. 76).

Technique

The arm is extended and the lateral edge of the biceps tendon at the level of the elbow is palpated. A skin wheal is made approximately halfway between this point and the lateral border of the arm. A 1 ½-inch, 23-gauge needle is inserted perpendicular to the skin and toward the humerus. Often a paresthesia of the radial nerve will be obtained; if so, 5 cc of local anesthetic is injected at this point. If the first attempt at eliciting a paresthesia is unsuccessful, fanwise movement of the needle tip will usually obtain one. Occasionally a paresthesia cannot be obtained, in which case the needle should be advanced to the bone and 7 to 10 cc of local anesthetic should be injected in several directions as the needle is withdrawn.

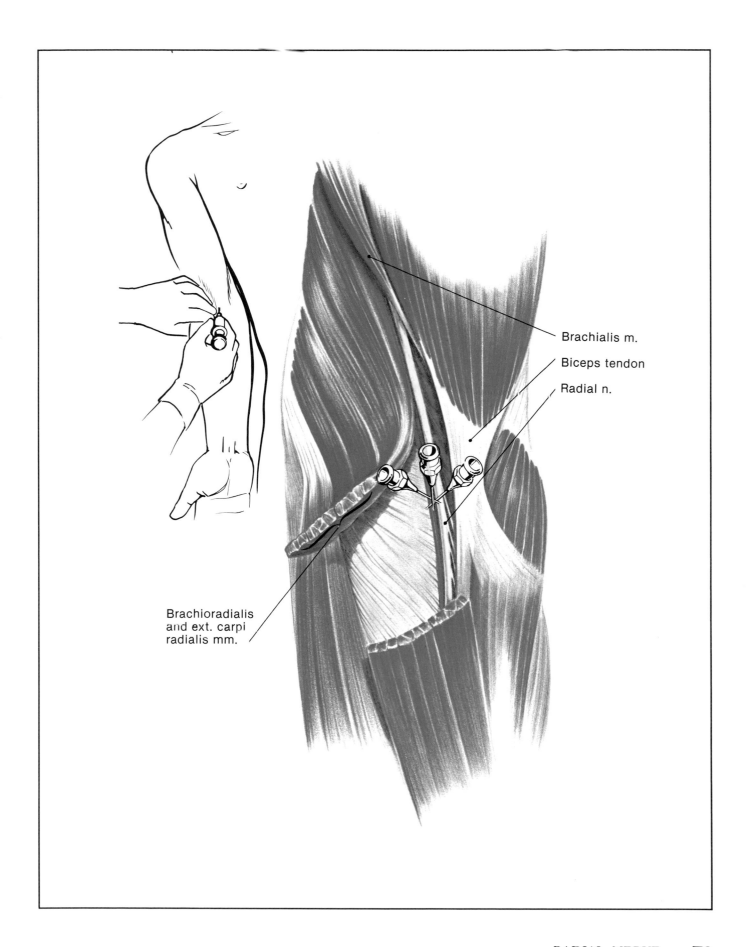

Brachialis m.

Biceps tendon

Radial n.

Brachioradialis
and ext. carpi
radialis mm.

Median Nerve

BLOCK AT THE ELBOW

Anatomy

The median nerve is formed by the fusion of lateral and median roots (see p. 62) and contains fibers from C5 through T1. It descends the arm with the brachial artery and at the level of the elbow is positioned just on its medial side. There are no branches of the nerve in the upper arm, but once in the forearm multiple branches are given off to flexor muscles. The median nerve enters the hand deep to the palmaris longus tendon, gives sensory branches to the palm, and ends in five digital cutaneous branches that supply the skin of the anterior surface of the outer three and a half fingers, as well as the skin over the dorsal terminal phalanges.

Technique

The arm is fully extended and the brachial artery is palpated in the crease of the anticubital fossa. A short-bevel, ½- to ¾-inch, 25-gauge needle is inserted just to the ulnar side of the artery. A paresthesia to the median nerve distribution in the hand is usually obtained at a depth of between ⅜ to ¾ inch below the skin level. Three to five cubic centimeters of anesthetic is injected.

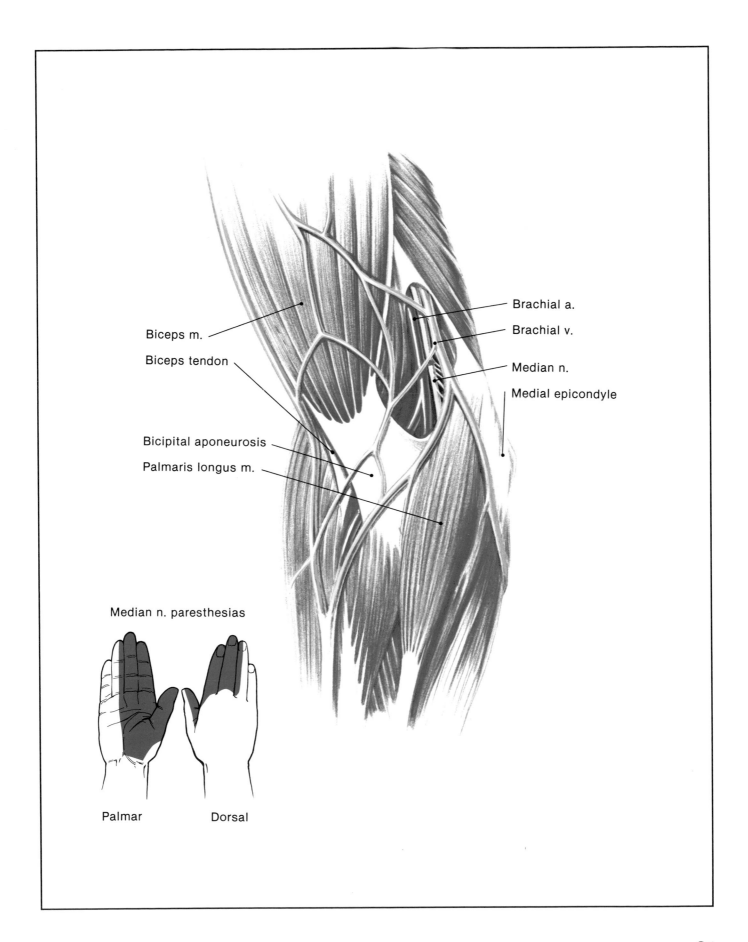

Biceps m.

Biceps tendon

Bicipital aponeurosis

Palmaris longus m.

Brachial a.

Brachial v.

Median n.

Medial epicondyle

Median n. paresthesias

Palmar   Dorsal

Ulnar Nerve

BLOCK AT THE ELBOW

Anatomy

The ulnar nerve is the main continuation of the medial cord. It descends in the arm accompanying the axillary artery and its continuation, the brachial artery. At about the midpoint of the upper arm it leaves the artery to move medially and lie between the prominences of the medial epicondyle and olecranon processes at the level of the elbow. Two cutaneous branches are given off: (1) the dorsal cutaneous branch, which supplies the ulnar side of the hand and the dorsum of the medial 1½ fingers, and (2) the palmar cutaneous branch, which provides some sensation to the ulnar side of the wrist and hand. In addition to several muscular branches, while in the hand its superficial terminal branch supplies the skin of the anterior medial 1½ fingers.

Technique

The patient's arm is flexed at the elbow and the olecranon process is identified. Between the olecranon process and the epicondyle of the humerus the ulnar nerve can usually be palpated through the skin. A ½- to ¾-inch block needle is inserted directly toward the nerve until a paresthesia is obtained. The needle is then withdrawn 1 mm and 8 to 10 cc of solution is slowly injected.

Note: Since the nerve is fairly well fixed with the arm in this position, it is not advised to inject if the patient has continued paresthesias.

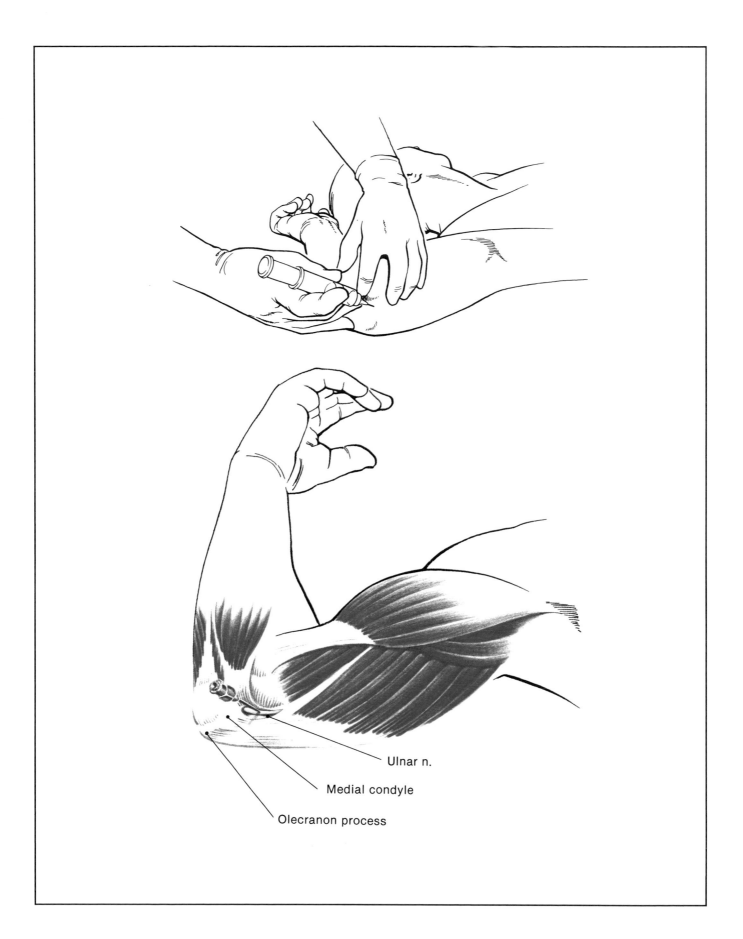

Ulnar n.

Medial condyle

Olecranon process

Radial Nerve

BLOCK AT THE WRIST

Anatomy

About two-thirds of the way down the forearm the radial nerve splits into various peripheral branches. One of the major branches of the nerve, at the level of the wrist, lies between the flexor carpi radialis and the radial artery. The other twigs spread out subcutaneously to innervate the dorsum of the hand.

Technique

The wrist is flexed slightly and the flexor carpi radialis is identified. A major peripheral branch of the radial nerve may be blocked by inserting a ½-inch, 25-gauge needle between the flexor carpi radialis and the radial artery and depositing 3 to 4 cc of local anesthetic.

Since other terminal branches course in the subcutaneous tissue along the dorsum of the wrist, however, a subcutaneous wheal of local anesthetic from the site of the first injection across the back of the wrist to just past the midline is required for complete anesthesia.

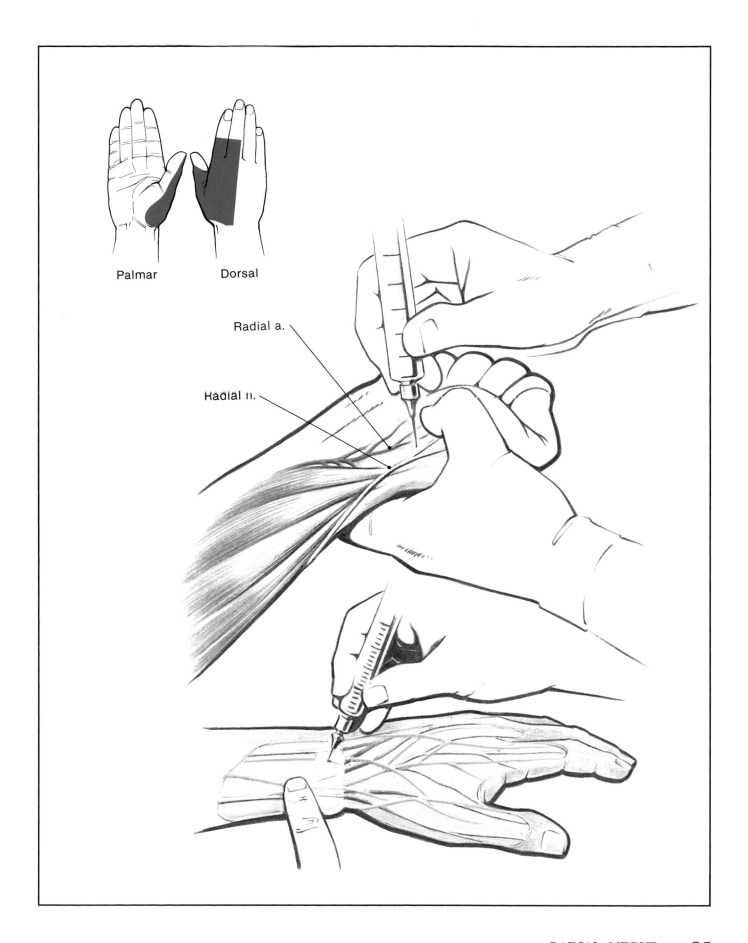

Palmar   Dorsal

Radial a.

Radial n.

Median Nerve

BLOCK AT THE WRIST

Anatomy

The median nerve lies deep to the palmaris longus tendon, between the tendons of the flexor digitorum superficialis and flexor carpi radialis at the level of the wrist.

Technique

The tendon of the palmaris longus is identified by having the patient flex the wrist against some resistance. A ½-inch, 25-gauge needle is inserted just medial and deep to the tendon, and 3 to 5 cc of local anesthetic is injected. Paresthesias may or may not be obtained.

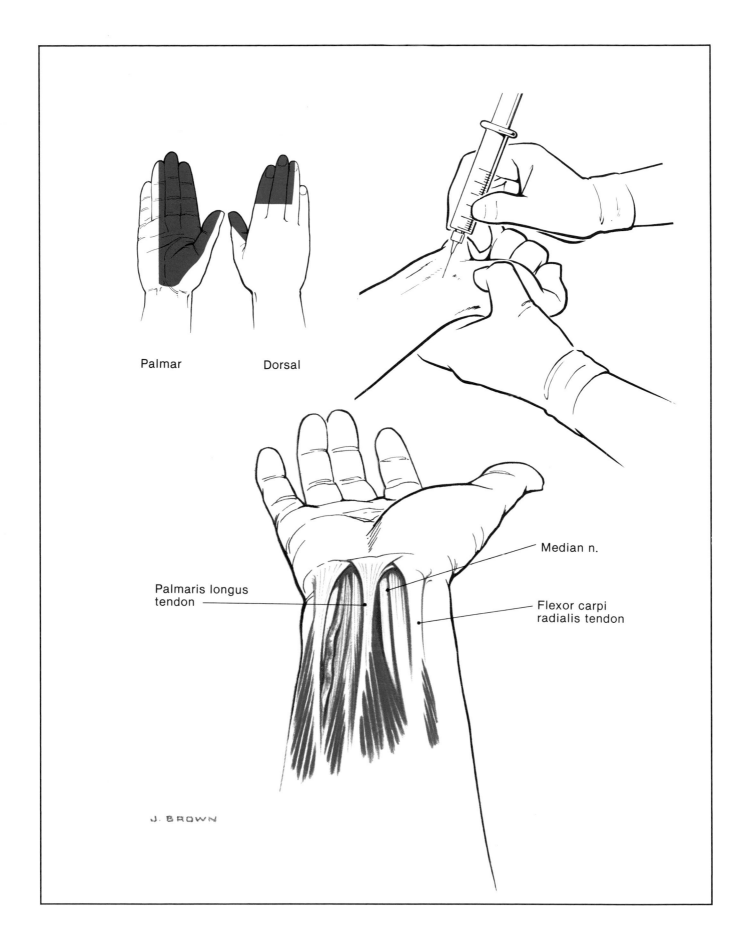

Palmar   Dorsal

Median n.

Palmaris longus
tendon

Flexor carpi
radialis tendon

J. BROWN

Ulnar Nerve

BLOCK AT THE WRIST

Anatomy

As it approaches the middle of the forearm the ulnar nerve lies between the flexor digitorum profundus and the flexor carpi ulnaris. In the lower portion of the forearm it gives off its two cutaneous branches (see p. 82). The ulnar nerve passes through the wrist on its way to innervate the structures of the hand between the tendon of the flexor carpi ulnaris and the ulnar artery.

Technique

The tendon of the flexor carpi ulnaris is identified by having the patient flex the wrist against mild resistance. On the lateral side of the tendon a ½- to ¾-inch block needle is inserted. Just deep to the tendon an ulnar paresthesia will be obtained. Three to five cubic centi- meters of solution is injected.

Note: If a paresthesia is not obtained with the first insertion of the needle, repeated fanned insertions will elicit one.

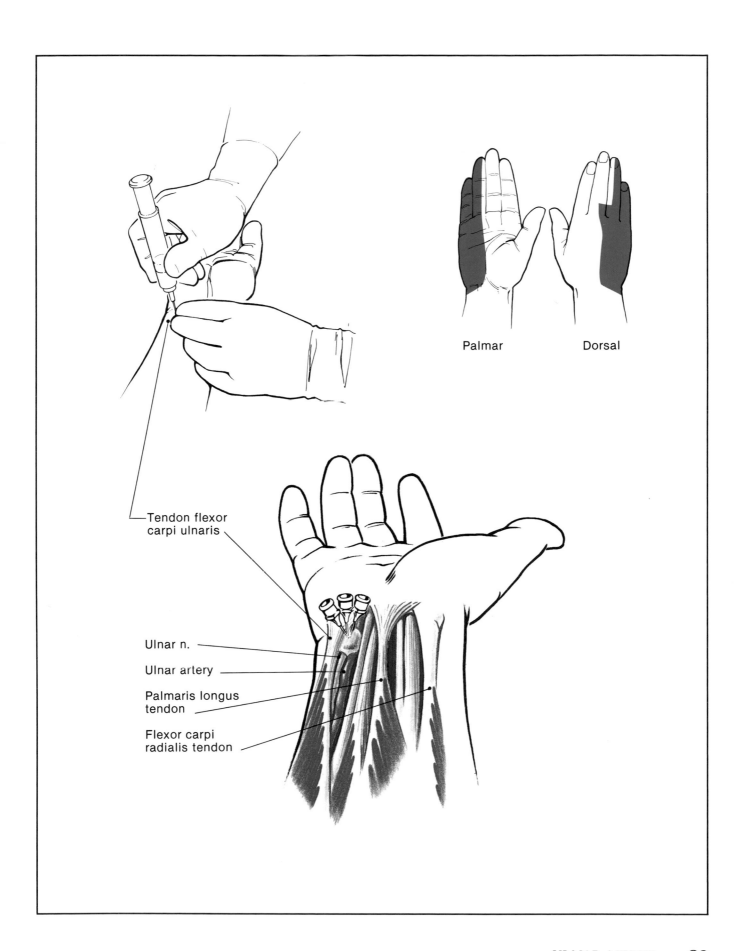

Palmar   Dorsal

Tendon flexor
carpi ulnaris

Ulnar n.

Ulnar artery

Palmaris longus
tendon

Flexor carpi
radialis tendon

Digital Nerve Blocks

COMMON DIGITAL NERVE BLOCK IN THE HAND (METACARPAL NERVE BLOCK)

Technique

For common digital nerve block in the hand a skin wheal is raised between the metacarpal bones on the dorsum of the hand. A 1-inch, 23-gauge block needle is inserted through it and 3 to 5 cc of local anesthetic is infiltrated as the needle is advanced slowly from the skin of the dorsum of the hand parallel to the metacarpal bone, stopping just short of the palmar surface. The common digital (metacarpal) nerve lies just above the flexor retinaculum of the hand, so most of the local anesthetic should be deposited close to the palmar surface.

COMMON DIGITAL NERVE BLOCK IN THE FOOT (METATARSAL NERVE BLOCK)

Technique

This block is the same as for the metacarpal block except that a longer needle (1½- to 2-inch) is required and 5 to 8 cc of local anesthetic is deposited between the metatarsal bones, most of it near the sole of the foot.

DIGITAL NERVE BLOCK—FINGER

Technique

The finger is supplied with four nerves, seen in a cross section view at approximately the 2-o'clock, 5-o'clock, 7-o'clock, and 10-o'clock positions. These nerves are blocked with small volumes of local anesthetic infiltrated between the skin and bone. A total of 3 cc injected slowly around the circumference of the finger at its base will provide adequate anesthesia. Epinephrine should not be used and paresthesias are not sought.

Note: Since mechanical compression of the vascular supply to the finger is possible, excessive volumes should not be used.

DIGITAL NERVE BLOCK—TOE

Technique

The procedure for the toe is exactly the same as for the finger except only 2 cc of solution is required.

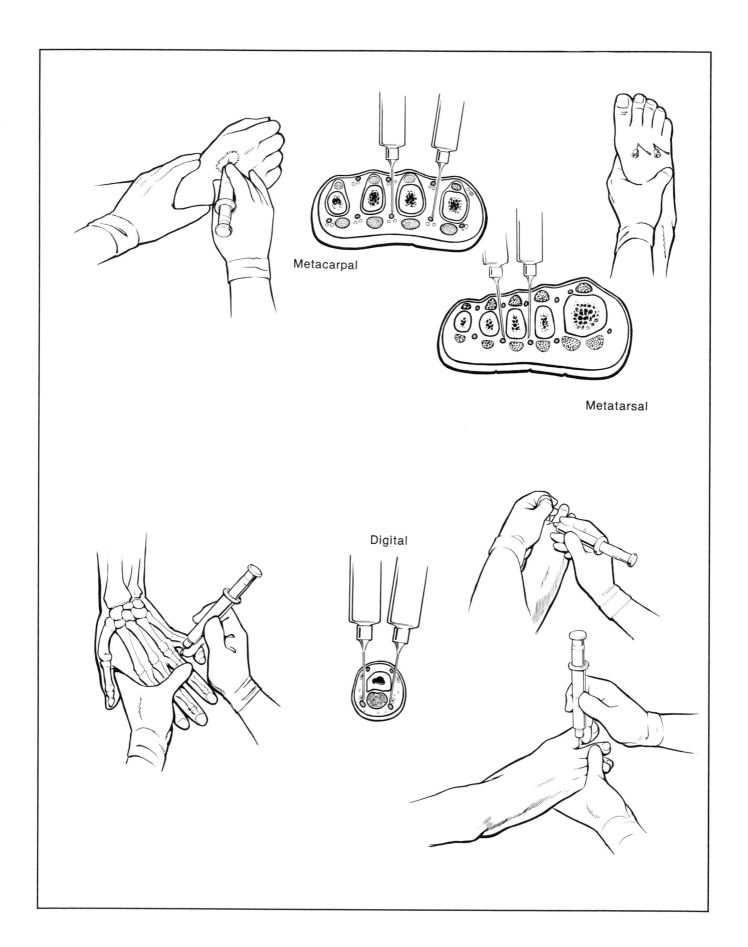

Metacarpal

Metatarsal

Digital

Thorax

Thoracic Paravertebral Nerve

Anatomy

The anatomy of the vertebral column is described in the section on spinal and epidural anesthesia (pp. 168–169). It is important to remember the relationship between the dorsal spine and the underlying vertebral body so that the correct thoracic paravertebral nerve can be approached.

Technique

For Mid-Thoracic Paravertebral Nerve Block. The patient can be positioned prone or laterally, with the affected side up. The prone position is preferred for both unilateral and bilateral block. The patient is positioned prone with a large, soft pillow under the chest. The dorsal spines are identified and the one immediately superior to the nerve to be blocked is noted. A skin wheal is made 1½ inches lateral to the spine, over the transverse process of the immediately inferior thoracic vertebrae. A 3-inch, 22-gauge block needle is inserted perpendicularly until the transverse process is contacted, at a depth of approximately 1½ inches. The needle is then withdrawn into the subcutaneous tissue and reinserted medially and inferiorly. When the needle is approximately an inch deeper than the transverse process a paresthesia of the thoracic nerve should be elicited. Five to eight cubic centimeters of local anesthetic is then injected.

If a paresthesia is not obtained as the needle is advanced, the needle will come in contact with the posterior lateral border of the vertebrae. If this happens the needle should be withdrawn into the subcutaneous tissue and redirected slightly more caudad or cephalad. If several insertions of the needle fail to produce a paresthesia and the bone of the vertebral body is repeatedly contacted, the needle should be withdrawn approximately ½ inch from the periosteum and 8 to 10 cc of local anesthetic infiltrated as the needle is very slowly withdrawn.

Note: Radiologic confirmation of needle placement is a great aid in performing this block. The proximity of the needle tip to the pleura and the epidural and intrathecal spaces necessitates great care when advancing the needle or injecting the solution.

Since a dural sleeve may persist into the paravertebral space, it is possible to inadvertently put local anesthetic directly into the cerebral spinal fluid. Aspiration may or may not reveal that the needle tip actually lies within the sleeve, so care must be exercised when making the injection.

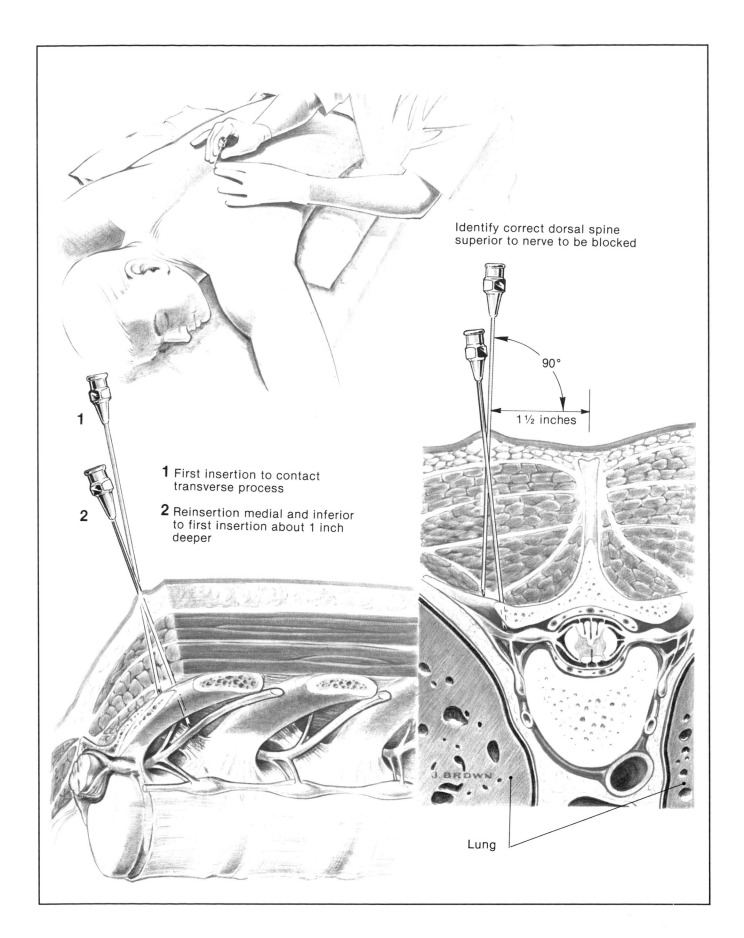

Identify correct dorsal spine superior to nerve to be blocked

90°

1 ½ inches

1 First insertion to contact transverse process

2 Reinsertion medial and inferior to first insertion about 1 inch deeper

J. BROWN

Lung

Splanchnic Nerve

Anatomy

There are usually three splanchnic nerves formed from thoracic sympathetic preganglionic fibers—the greater, lesser, and least splanchnic nerves. The greater splanchnic nerve originates primarily from sympathetic filaments arising from T7, T8, and T9. However, fibers can come from as high as T3 or as low as T10. Individual roots tend to migrate to the inferior lateral surface of the vertebrae, where they fuse at approximately the T9 to T10 level. The nerve pierces the diaphragm, then separates again into multiple fibers that terminate in the celiac ganglia.

The lesser splanchnic nerve is formed from T11 and occasionally T12 preganglionic fibers, and lies several millimeters above the greater splanchnic nerve, between it and the sympathetic chain ganglia. After passing through the diaphragm the lesser splanchnic nerve's terminal fibers fuse with those of the greater splanchnic nerve to end in the celiac ganglia. In addition, the lesser splanchnic nerve contributes some fibers to the preaortic sympathetic plexus.

The least splanchnic nerve usually arises from T12 and is a rather small filament that pierces through the abdomen with the other splanchnic nerves, ending in the preaortic ganglia. Occasionally there is also an accessory splanchnic nerve from T12 that follows the same course as the least splanchnic nerve.

Technique

The patient lies prone with a pillow under the upper abdomen. At a point 3 inches lateral to the spinous process of L1 and just under the margin of the twelfth rib a skin wheal is raised. After adequately infiltrating the soft tissue in the general direction of the needle path with local anesthetic, a 4- to 6-inch, 22-gauge block needle is inserted until it contacts the transverse process of L1. This should occur at a depth of approximately 1½ to 2 inches. The needle is then withdrawn and redirected superiorly and medially to contact the body of the T12 vertebrae. The depth of the needle should be noted. The needle is withdrawn into the subcutaneous tissue and the angle made with the skin lessened. It is then reinserted and advanced to the anterior lateral surface of the T12 vertebrae, where the nerves lie. Eight to ten cubic centimeters of local anesthetic is injected.

Note: Radiologic confirmation of needle position is a great aid in performing this block. The procedure must be done bilaterally to achieve any efficacy whatsoever. It should be noted that for almost all indications block of the celiac plexus is just as effective.

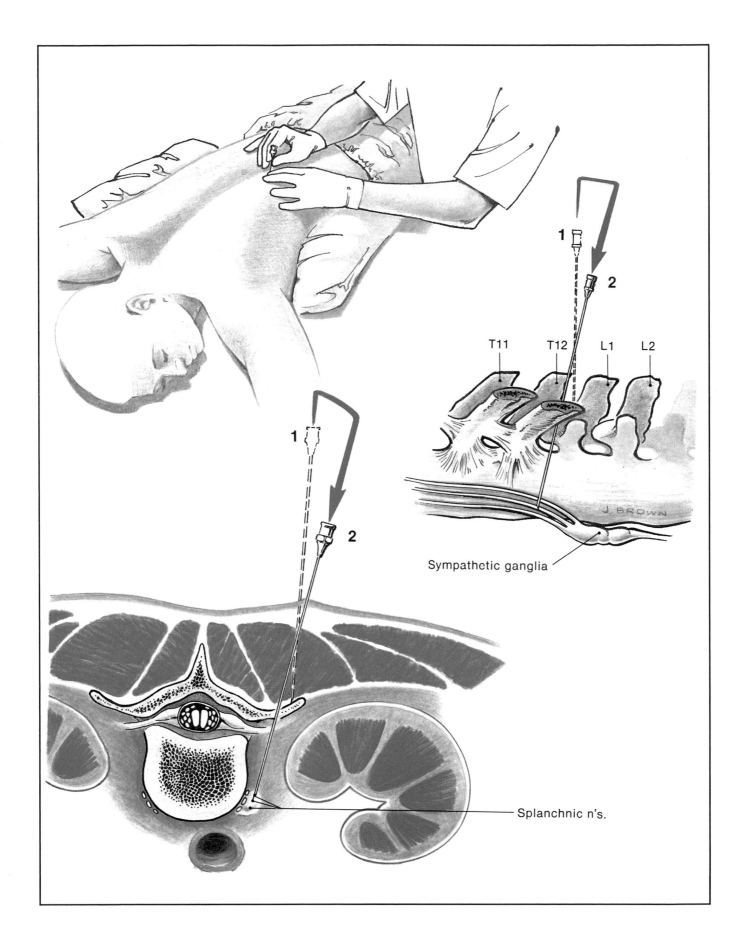

T11 T12 L1 L2

Sympathetic ganglia

Splanchnic n's.

J. BROWN

Thoracic Sympathetic Ganglion

Anatomy

The preganglionic fibers of the sympathetic outflow originate in the intermediolateral horn of the gray matter of the spinal cord. They exit the vertebral foramen accompanying the anterior root of a thoracic nerve. Just beyond the foramen the sympathetic fibers go ventrally via the white rami communicantes to the ganglia of the sympathetic chain. Some of the sympathetic outflow ends in the segmental ganglion anastomosing with postganglionic fibers there. Others pass directly through the ganglion, still as preganglionic fibers, ending in the colateral ganglia.

Within the sympathetic segmental ganglia, preganglionic and postganglionic fibers synapse. Some of the postsynaptic nerves return to their respective segmental nerves via the gray rami communicantes innervating blood vessels, sweat glands, and the pilomotor muscles of the skin. Other postganglionic fibers may run 3 to 6 dermatomes caudad or cephalad through the sympathetic trunks to terminate in more distal ganglia. Still others pass through the vertebral ganglia to end in a variety of nerve plexi, such as the cardiac plexus and the hypogastric plexus.

The position of the sympathetic ganglia vary depending on the anatomic level of the spinal cord where they are found. The first thoracic sympathetic ganglion becomes fused with the lower cervical ganglion to form the inferior pole of the stellate ganglion. In general, as one descends from T2 to L2 the site of the ganglia move from just beneath the rib to the anterior lateral surface of the vertebrae. The second thoracic ganglion lies just anterior to the medial portion of the neck of the rib. The next three or four ganglia lie in front of the corresponding head of the rib. The lower thoracic ganglia from T7 to T10 are located just below the rib along the posterior superior surface of the vertebrae. T11 and T12 ganglia are on the lateral surface of the vertebrae, approximately, whereas the lumbar ganglia move progressively more toward the anterior lateral surface.

Technique

The upper and middle thoracic ganglia lie in close proximity to the somatic nerves. They will almost always be blocked when a thoracic paravertebral nerve block is successful. The technique for block of the upper ganglia is therefore the same as noted for thoracic paravertebral nerve block. (p. 94).

For the middle and lower thoracic ganglia the needle should be advanced past the somatic nerve to touch the lateral body of the vertebrae. Five cubic centimeters of local anesthetic should then be injected.

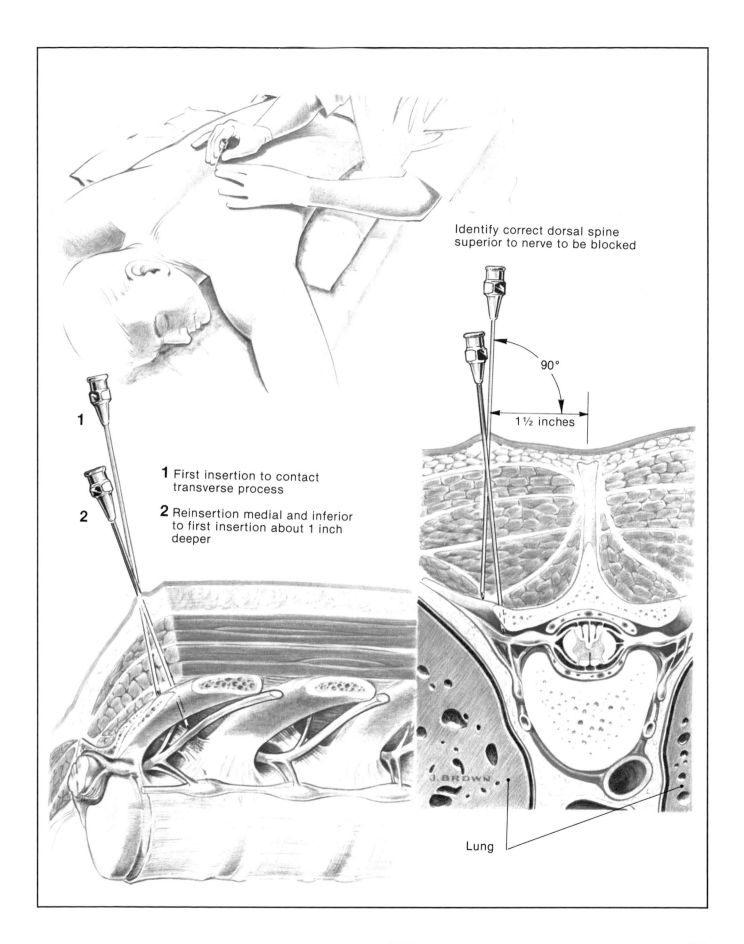

Identify correct dorsal spine
superior to nerve to be blocked

90°

1½ inches

1 First insertion to contact
transverse process

2 Reinsertion medial and inferior
to first insertion about 1 inch
deeper

J. BROWN

Lung

Intercostal Nerves

UNILATERAL BLOCK

Anatomy

Intercostal nerves are the fusion of dorsal and ventral roots that attach to the cord as a series of fine rootlets. Dorsal rootlets are actually nerve extensions from the dorsal ganglion, which is located at the intervertebral foramen. Just distal to the ganglion the dorsal root is joined by the now-fused rootlets of the ventral root to form the peripheral nerve. The dural covering surrounding the roots becomes continuous with the epineurium of the nerve. After the anterior and posterior roots of the nerves fuse, a small recurrent branch, called the meningeal nerve, returns through the foramen to supply a segment of the meninges and corresponding vertebrae. Immediately after leaving the foramen a posterior ramus is given off. This provides sensation to the midline structures of the back. Almost at the same level, the rami communicantes leave in a ventral direction to join the sympathetic chain ganglion. As the nerve courses to the periphery at about the level of the midaxillary line, its lateral branch arises. It in turn divides into a posterior and anterior division, supplying the skin over the back and anterior body surface, respectively. The nerve then continues to the front of the body, where its anterior cutaneous branch supplies the midline skin and soft tissues.

The anatomic position of the nerve in relation to the spine and rib is of importance. The fused nerve exits the intervertebral foramen and goes between the pleura and posterior intercostal membrane. Deep to the rib and about 3 cm distal to the foramen the nerve pierces the posterior intercostal membrane to enter the subcostal groove, becoming part of the neurovascular complex. It reenters the intercostal space between the ribs somewhat medial to the anterior axillary line. Since the subcostal groove no longer exists at this point, the nerve lies in the substance of the internal intercostal muscle. It eventually goes beneath the muscle to run next to the pleura, with its terminal end just anterior to the internal mammary artery. The final sensory fibers of the nerve across the midline provide innervation to about ½ to 1 inch of the contralateral side of the body.

Described above is the typical course of the second to sixth intercostal nerves. The first thoracic nerve is somewhat different in anatomy. Its anterior division divides into large superior and small inferior branches. The superior branch enters the groove between the scalene muscles and becomes part of the lower trunk of the brachial plexus. The smaller branch continues in the intercostal space, where it sends a contribution to the intercostobrachial nerve.

The seventh through eleventh thoracic nerves run courses similar to those described above until they come to the anterior margin of the ribs. At this point they pass underneath the costal cartilages and into the space between the transverse abdominal and internal oblique muscles. At the lateral margin of the rectus muscle the nerves pierce the posterior sheath and run within the muscle. Near the midline they go through the anterior rectus sheath and proceed subcutaneously to the midline, giving off many cutaneous branches.

The T12 nerve is unique in that it gives off a branch to join the first lumbar nerve before going laterally. It pierces the transverse abdominal muscle to lie between it and the internal oblique muscle. Branches from the lateral cutaneous portion of the twelfth nerve supply sensation to the skin overlying the hip joint.

Technique

The patient is positioned semiprone with the side to be blocked uppermost. The arm is raised above the head in order to elevate the scapula. The appropriate rib or ribs are identified by counting up from the T12 rib or down from the cervical area.

The thumb and index finger bracket the rib. This should be done at the point between the posterior axillary line and costal angle where the rib is easiest to palpate. A ¾- to 1 ½-inch, 22-gauge needle can be used for the majority of cases; for a very obese or thickly muscled patient a longer needle might be re-quired. The needle is directed between the fingers at the lower portion of the rib at an angle of approximately 20 degrees cephalad. The rib is contacted and the depth noted. The soft tissue and needle tip are retracted inferiorly, with the needle keeping intermittent contact with the surface of the rib. The operator will feel the needle tip leave the inferior edge of the rib. It should then be advanced 2 to 3 mm, so that the tip rests near the subcostal groove. Three to four cubic centimeters of local anesthetic is injected.

1 Palpate correct rib with thumb and forefinger

2 Insert needle approx. 20° cephalad through skin wheal placed over lower border of rib

3 At rib's undersurface advance needle 2 mm

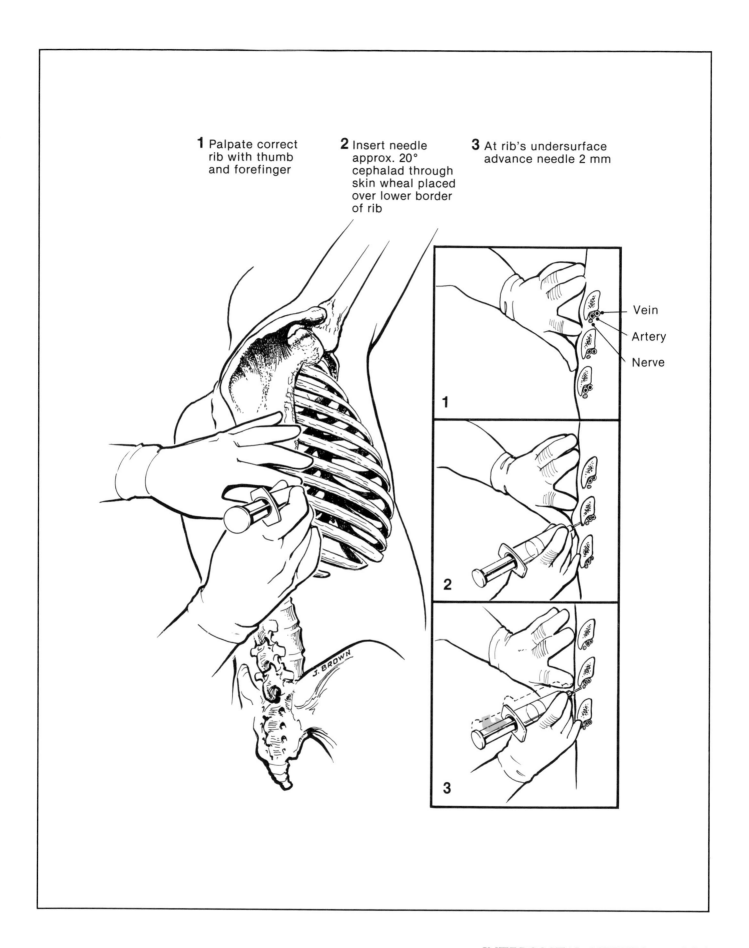

Vein

Artery

Nerve

J. BROWN

Intercostal Nerves

BILATERAL BLOCK

Anatomy

See anatomy for Intercostal Nerves—Unilateral Block (p. 100).

Technique

The patient is placed in the prone position, both arms raised above the head. Past this point the technique is the same as for the unilateral block (p. 100). Occasionally it may be necessary to do the block with the patient in less than optimal position. For such a case put the patient in a 45 degree prone position. Although slightly more difficult from a technical standpoint, this technique can be successfully used to perform bilateral blocks.

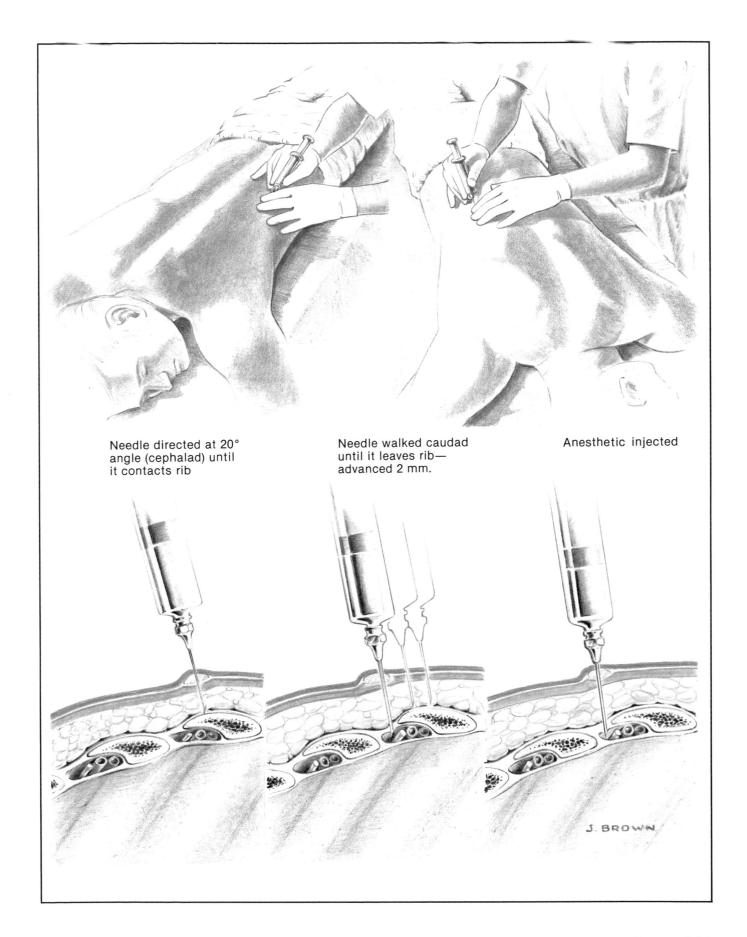

Needle directed at 20° angle (cephalad) until it contacts rib

Needle walked caudad until it leaves rib— advanced 2 mm.

Anesthetic injected

J. BROWN

Breast

Anatomy

The breast is innervated by mammary rami from the third through sixth or seventh intercostal nerves. In addition, some superficial terminal branches from the cervical plexus may provide sensation to the skin over the anterior part of the apex of the breast.

Technique

The innervation to the breast can be blocked by running a wheal of local anesthetic in the subcutaneous tissue above the apex of the breast, then down its lateral border and inferiorly in the retromammary space. About 15 to 20 cc of a dilute local anesthetic solution with epinephrine 1:200,000 is used.

Block of the breast can also be accomplished by blocking the T3 to T7 intercostal nerves. This should be supplemented by a subcutaneous infiltration just above the apex of the breast to block the descending superficial fibers from the cervical plexus.

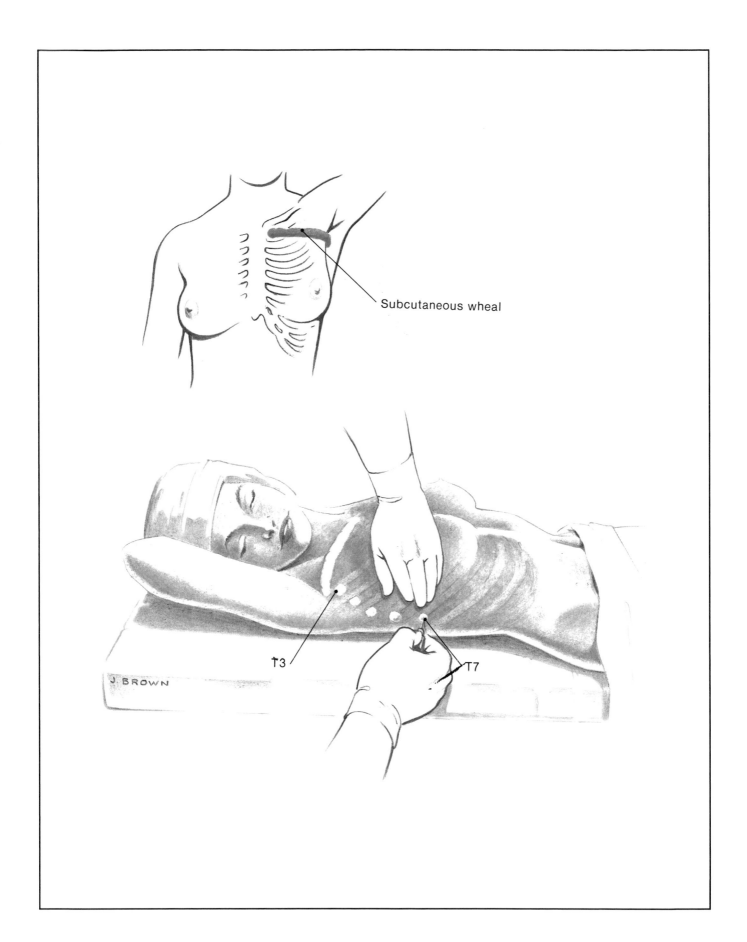

Subcutaneous wheal

T3

T7

J. BROWN

Abdomen

Lumbar Somatic Nerves

Anatomy

The anatomy of the vertebral column is reviewed on page 168. The lumbar somatic nerves get progressively larger from L1 to L5. The upper three lumbar primary ventral rami, together with part of the fourth root, form the lumbar plexus. The remainder of L4 joins the fifth root to become the lumbar contribution to the sacral plexus.

The spine of the lumbar vertebrae lies immediately above its corresponding vertebral body. Its caudad tip is parallel to the cephalad edge of the transverse process of the next lower vertebrae. The lumbar nerve exits from the spinal canal via the intervertebral foramen and is about 1 inch deep to the caudal edge of the transverse process.

Immediately after the nerve exits the foramen it gives off a posterior primary division that provides sensation to the midline structures of the back, and an anterior primary division that becomes part of the lumbar or sacral plexus.

Technique

The patient lies on the side opposite the one to be blocked. The correct dorsal spine is identified by either counting up from the sacrum, noting the line between the iliac crests (should be at the level of L4 spine), or counting down from T12. A skin wheal is made 1 ½ to 2 inches laterally to the inferior tip of the dorsal spine, and a 3- to 4-inch, 22-gauge block needle inserted perpendicularly after generous infiltration with local anesthetic. The transverse process of the vertebra immediately below is contacted. The needle is then withdrawn to the subcutaneous tissue and reinserted to pass superior to the transverse process in a slightly medial direction. At an additional depth of about 1 inch a paresthesia should be elicited. If not the needle should be reinserted until one is obtained.

If several attempts are not successful in evoking a paresthesia the needle is again inserted to a depth of about 1 inch past the transverse process, where 10 cc of local anesthetic is infiltrated as the needle is moved in several directions. If a paresthesia is obtained, 5 to 8 cc will produce an adequate block.

Note: If neurolytic agents are used the procedure should be done with x-ray verification of needle-tip placement. Obtaining a paresthesia is more important in such cases.

Note: If the block is to be done bilaterally the patient should be positioned prone with a soft pillow placed under the abdomen. The procedure is then done exactly as described above.

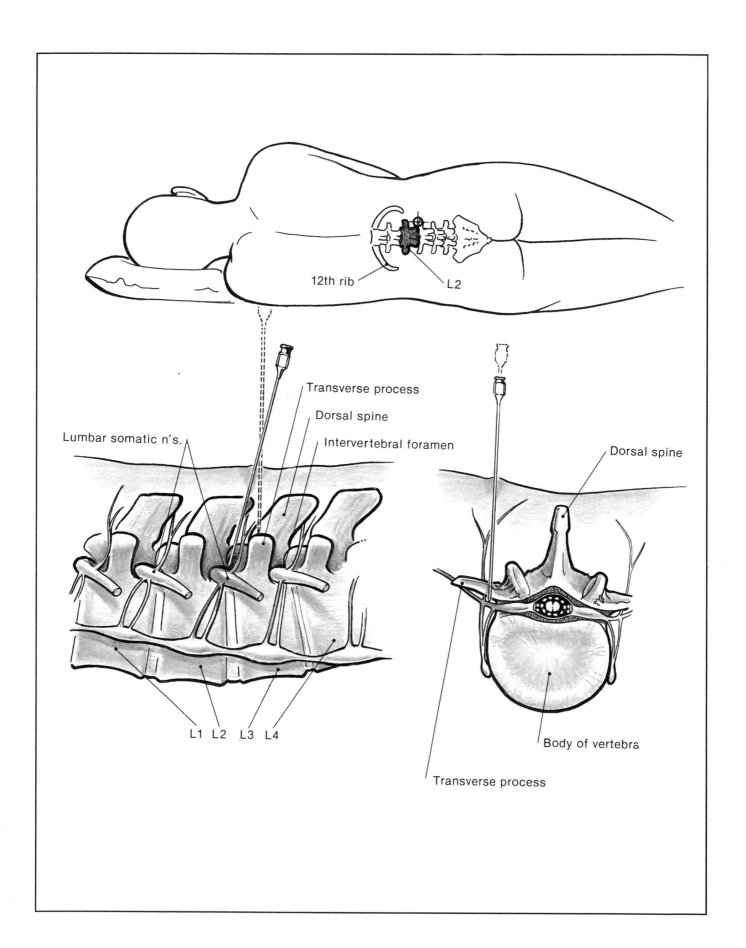

12th rib

L2

Transverse process

Dorsal spine

Intervertebral foramen

Lumbar somatic n's.

L1 L2 L3 L4

Dorsal spine

Body of vertebra

Transverse process

Lumbar Sympathetic Ganglion

Anatomy

The lumbar sympathetic ganglia are a continuation of the sympathetic chain that originates in the thoracic region (see p. 98). The sympathetic ganglia in the lumbar region lie along the anterior lateral surface of the vertebral bodies. Postganglionic fibers either return to their corresponding lumbar nerve via the gray rami communicantes, go to the aortic and hypogastric plexi, or accompany blood vessels of the abdomen and extremities. The L1 ganglion also sends fibers to the celiac plexus.

The majority of the sympathetic outflow to an extremity passes through L2, L3, and L4 paravertebral lumbar ganglia.

Technique

The patient is positioned as for a lumbar somatic nerve block and the appropriate dorsal spine is identified (see p. 108). A 4-inch, 22-gauge block needle is used. The superior edge of the dorsal spine is identified and a skin wheal is made 3 inches lateral to it. After generously infiltrating the soft tissue, the needle is advanced slightly medially toward the body of the vertebra. The needle will first contact the transverse process of the vertebra, usually at a depth of from 1½ to 2 inches. The needle is then redirected slightly caudad and medially and advanced until the body of the vertebra is contacted. This should be at an additional depth of from 1 to 1½ inches. The angle the needle makes with the skin is then lessened to allow the needle to go ½ to ¾ inch past the lateral edge of the body of the vertebra. Five to eight cubic centimeters of local anesthetic is injected. No paresthesias are sought.

Note: Additional verification of position can be made by noting a subtle loss of resistance to ballottement of an air-filled syringe attached to the block needle. Resistance will decrease as the needle pierces the psoas muscle to enter the groove between the psoas and the vertebral body where the ganglion lies.

Note: X-ray verification of needle position is helpful in the performance of this block and becomes of extreme importance if neurolytic solutions are used.

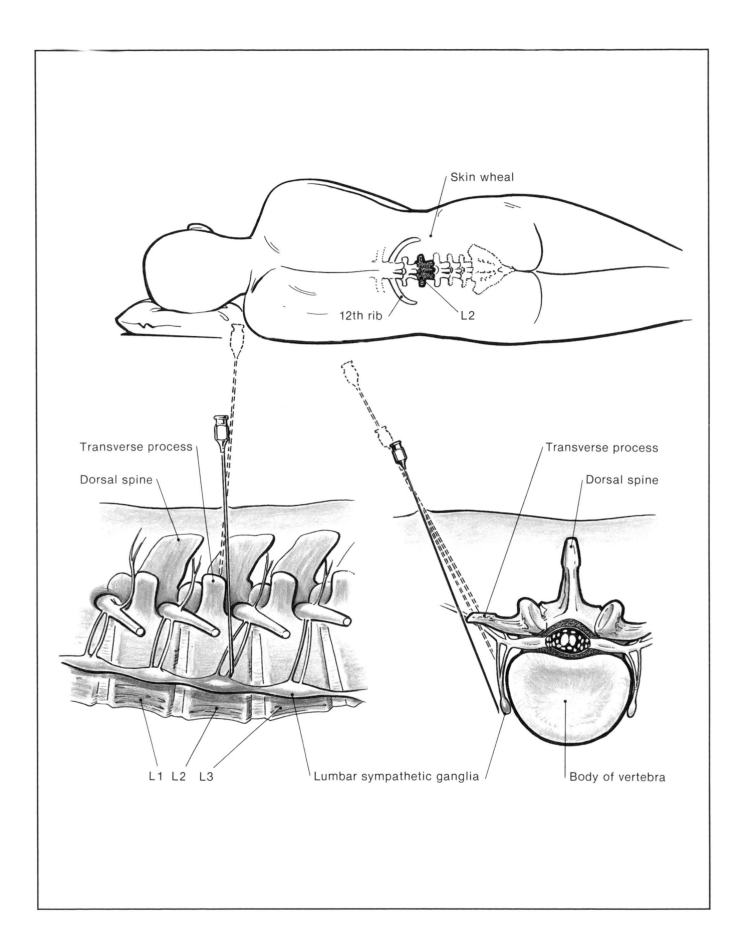

Skin wheal

12th rib

L2

Transverse process

Dorsal spine

Transverse process

Dorsal spine

L1 L2 L3

Lumbar sympathetic ganglia

Body of vertebra

Celiac Plexus

Anatomy

The celiac plexus is the fusion of the two celiac ganglia with several smaller ganglia found in the region of the celiac arterial trunk. It usually exists as two large masses lying on either side of the aorta at the origin of the celiac artery, although many variations of this structure exist.

The plexus receives both afferent and efferent nerve input. The efferent fibers arise from (1) the greater and lesser splanchnic nerves bilaterally, (2) postganglionic fibers from the upper lumbar sympathetic ganglia, and (3) terminal branches of both vagus nerves. Afferent fibers are both sympathetic and parasympathetic in origin. Parasympathetic fibers start in the viscera and ascend through the celiac plexus to the esophageal plexi. Sympathetic fibers also originate in the viscera and pass through the celiac plexus to the chain ganglia or splanchnic nerves on their way to the spinal cord.

The dimensions of the celiac plexus are quite variable. Generally the plexus is 1 to 1½ inches long and 1 to 2 inches wide. It surrounds the celiac artery, which is at the level of the first lumbar vertebrae, just anterior to the crura of the diaphragm. The right and left celiac ganglia are the largest components of the plexus. Each is approximately 2 to 3 mm thick and connected to the other by numerous fibers.

Technique

The patient is positioned prone, arms abducted to slightly greater than 90 degrees and bent at the elbow for comfort. The inferior border of the left 12th rib is outlined and the dorsal spine of L1 identified. At a point 3 to 4 inches lateral to the inferior margin of the L1 spine and just beneath the lower border of the 12th rib a 4- to 6-inch, 22-gauge block needle is inserted at an angle of 30 to 45 degrees toward the body of the L1 vertebra. The intended needle path should be generously infiltrated with local anesthetic. As the needle is advanced, the transverse process of L1 should be contacted at a depth of approximately 1½ inches. The needle is then withdrawn into the subcutaneous tissue and redirected to pass either superior or inferior to the transverse process and toward the body of the vertebra. Once the body of the vertebra is contacted and the depth of the needle noted, the needle is withdrawn again into the subcutaneous tissue. The angle previously made with the skin is decreased so that the tip of the needle passes the lateral edge of the body of L1. It is then advanced approximately 1 inch, at which point it should lie just deep to the anterior surface. After careful aspiration to ensure that the needle has not inadvertently entered the aorta or other major vessel, 30 to 50 cc of a dilute local anesthetic is injected.

Note: This procedure is best performed under x-ray guidance so the relationship of the tip of the needle and the bony structures is known at all times. Although the block may be performed from either side, the left side is preferred. This is because the vena cava, a major vascular structure that must be avoided, runs just to the right of the midline in the area of the block.

Note: The block may also be performed with the patient in the lateral position.

Note: Although some advise a bilateral approach when neurolytic solutions are used, the technique described above will suffice in the majority of cases.

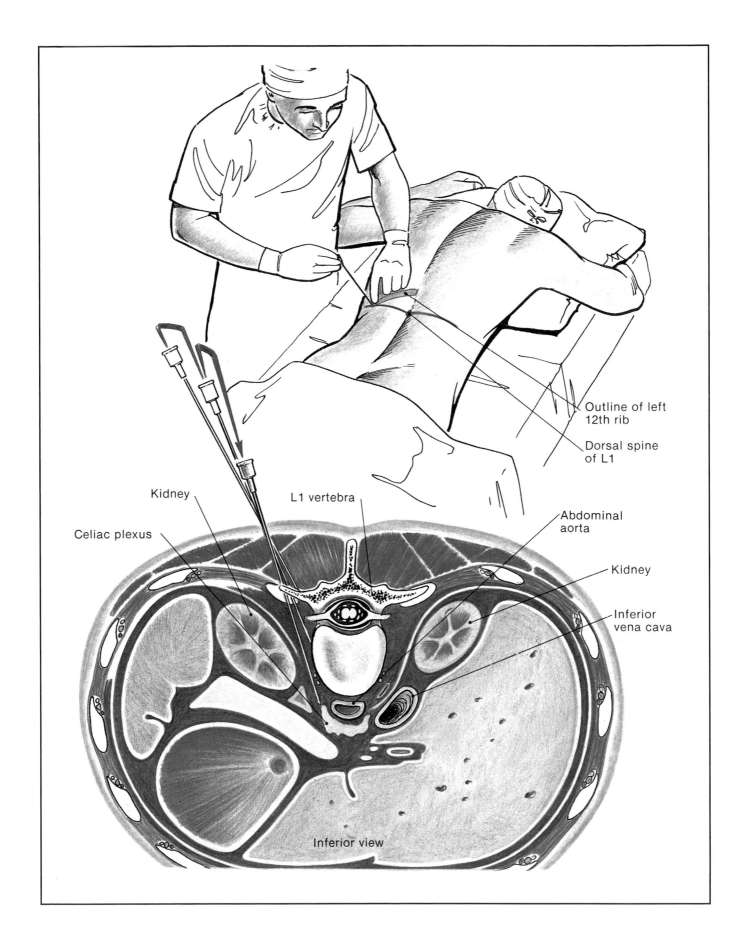

Outline of left
12th rib

Dorsal spine
of L1

Kidney

L1 vertebra

Celiac plexus

Abdominal
aorta

Kidney

Inferior
vena cava

Inferior view

Ilioinguinal and Iliohypogastric Nerves

Anatomy

Both the ilioinguinal and iliohypogastric nerves originate from the L1 nerve root. There may also be a small contribution from T12. The iliohypogastric nerve courses around the body and at the level of the iliac crest perforates the posterior part of the transverse abdominal muscle to lie between it and the external oblique muscle. There it divides into lateral and anterior cutaneous branches. The lateral branch pierces both the internal and external oblique muscles immediately above the iliac crest, providing sensation to the skin of the posterior lateral gluteal region. The anterior branch pierces the internal oblique muscle approximately 1 inch medial to the anterior superior spine. It then perforates the external oblique muscle and sends sensory fibers to the skin of the abdomen above the pubis.

The ilioinguinal nerve, which is usually somewhat smaller than the iliohypogastric nerve, perforates the transverse abdominal muscle at the level of the iliac crest, where it occasionally anastomoses with branches of the iliohypogastric nerve. It then pierces the internal oblique muscle and accompanies the spermatic chord through the inguinal ring and into the inguinal canal. It provides sensation to the superior inner aspect of the thigh, the skin over the root of the penis and upper part of the scrotum in the male, and the skin covering the mons pubis and lateral part of labia in the female.

Technique

About 1 inch medial to the anterior superior iliac spine and on a line between the spine and the umbilicus a ¾- to 1½-inch needle is inserted and 8 to 10 cc of local anesthetic is deposited as the needle pierces the fascias of the oblique muscles. Since this point is sometimes difficult to determine, fanwise and up-and-down infiltration of local anesthetic is required for a successful block.

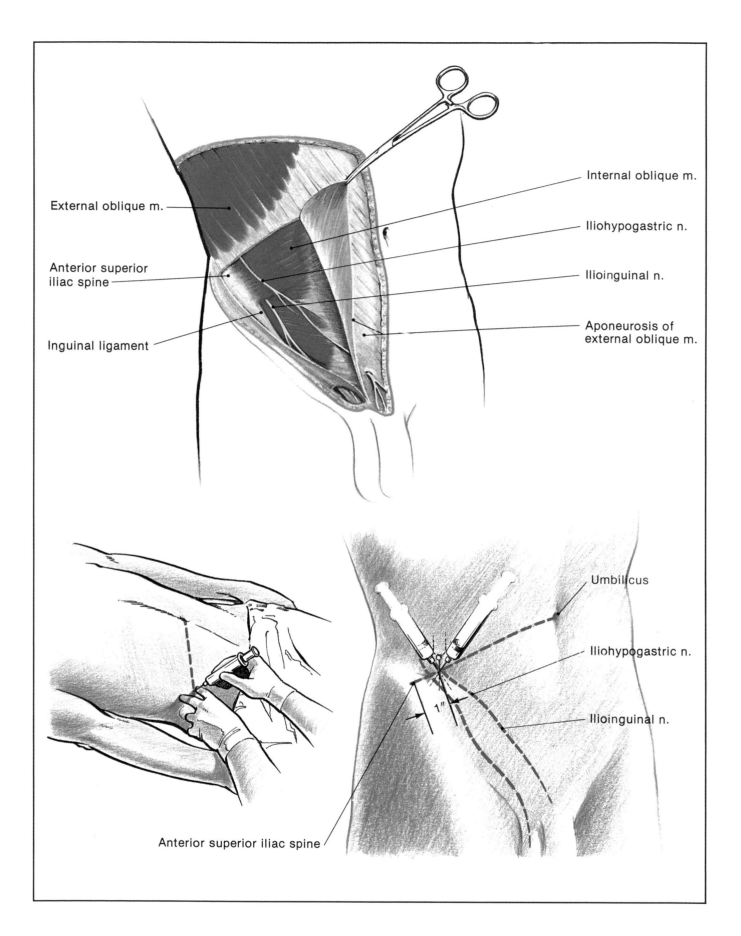

External oblique m.

Anterior superior iliac spine

Inguinal ligament

Internal oblique m.

Iliohypogastric n.

Ilioinguinal n.

Aponeurosis of external oblique m.

Anterior superior iliac spine

Umbilicus

Iliohypogastric n.

Ilioinguinal n.

1"

Genitofemoral Nerve

Anatomy

The genitofemoral nerve arises from the first and second lumbar nerves. After passing through the psoas muscle it divides into femoral and genital branches. The femoral branch joins with the femoral artery to go underneath the inguinal ligament and supply a small area of skin immediately below it. In the male the genital branch runs with the spermatic cord to supply the cremaster and dartos muscles and sends small terminal sensory fibers to the skin of the scrotum. In the female it runs in the inguinal canal with terminal fibers going to the round ligament of the uterus and the skin of the labium majus.

Technique

The terminal branches of the genital division are blocked by spreading 2 to 3 cc of local anesthetic through a 1-inch, 22-gauge block needle in the soft tissue down through the inguinal ligament just lateral to the pubic spine.

The terminal fibers of the femoral branch are blocked by infiltrating subcutaneously just below the middle third of the inguinal ligament with 3 to 5 cc of local anesthetic.

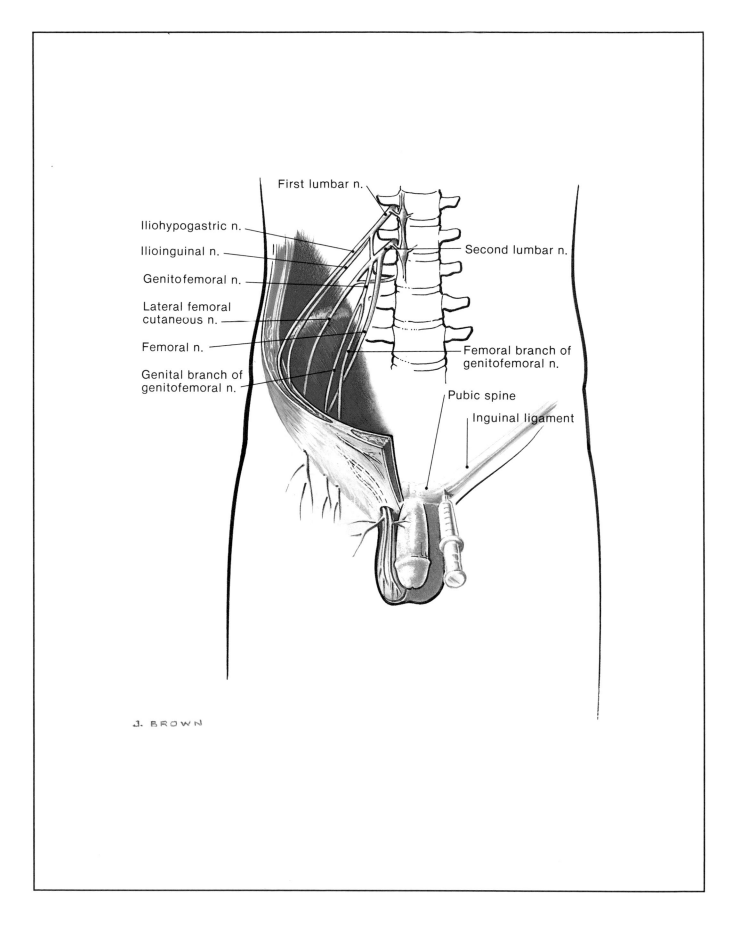

First lumbar n.

Iliohypogastric n.

Ilioinguinal n.

Genitofemoral n.

Lateral femoral cutaneous n.

Femoral n.

Genital branch of genitofemoral n.

Second lumbar n.

Femoral branch of genitofemoral n.

Pubic spine

Inguinal ligament

J. BROWN

Abdominal Field Block

Anatomy

Anatomic paths of the intercostal nerves have been described on page 100. These nerves supply sensory innervation to the overlying abdominal skin, motor fibers to the abdominal muscles, and sensation to the underlying parietal pleura.

Technique

Skin wheals are raised along the terminations of the ribs from T7 through T11. Local anesthetic is then infiltrated connecting the skin wheals and deep to the costal margins. The wall of anesthetic goes from the T11 tip of the rib centrally along the costal margin to the xiphoid process. If the procedure to be undertaken crosses the midline of the body, repeat the above steps on the contralateral side. If limited to one side, subcutaneous infiltration of local anesthetic should be continued from the xiphoid process to the umbilicus.

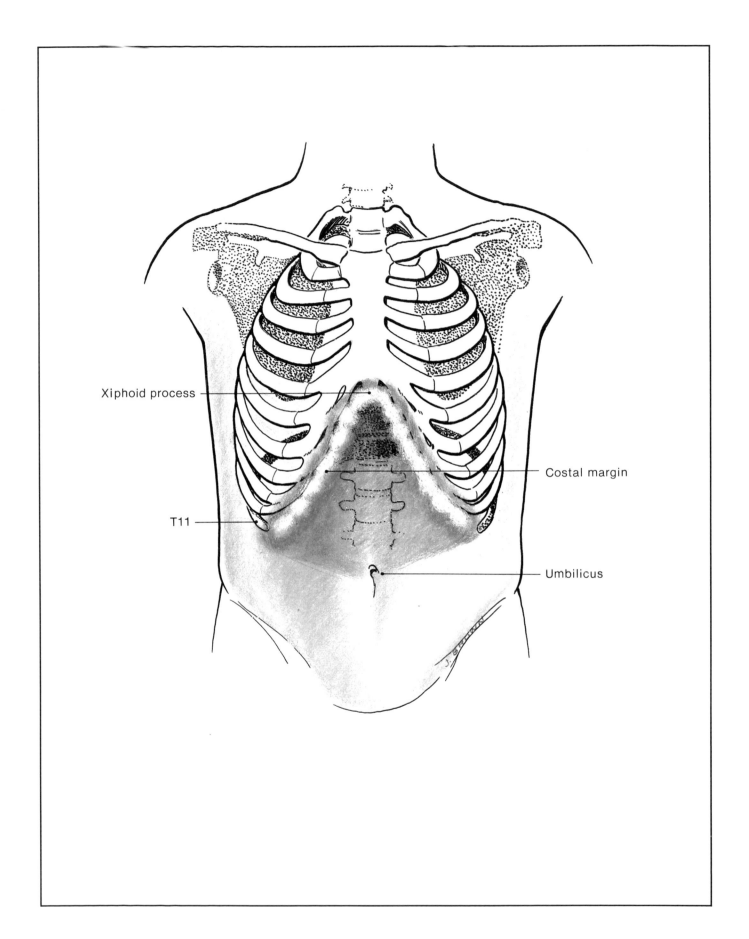

Xiphoid process

Costal margin

T11

Umbilicus

Inguinal Region

Anatomy

The inguinal region receives most of its sensory innervation via the ilioinguinal and iliohypogastric nerves. These are both primarily L1 in origin. Minor contributions may also be made from T12, L2, and the genitofemoral nerve. (For anatomy of the ilioinguinal and iliohypogastric nerves see p. 114; for the genitofemoral nerve see p. 116).

Technique

The ilioinguinal and iliohypogastric nerves are blocked as described on page 114. Following this, a 3- to 4-inch, 22-gauge needle is inserted through the same area as the initial insertion and advanced on a line between the anterior superior iliac spine and the umbilicus. Approximately 20 cc of local anesthetic is infiltrated into the soft tissue as the needle is advanced. This will block the terminal branches of T12 and perhaps T11 as they course toward the midline of the body.

In a similar manner a 3-inch block needle is inserted between the anterior superior iliac spine and the pubic spine, again infiltrating local anesthetic in the soft tissue. An additional 20 cc of local anesthetic may be required to adequately infiltrate this tissue.

This will produce skin anesthesia for surgical incision. If the spermatic cord is to be manipulated, infiltration of 2 to 3 cc of local anesthetic around the cord at the internal ring will complete the anesthesia.

Note: Some advise infiltration directly over a hernia skin incision. This should be unnecessary, however, if adequate block of the ilioinguinal and iliohypogastric nerves is achieved.

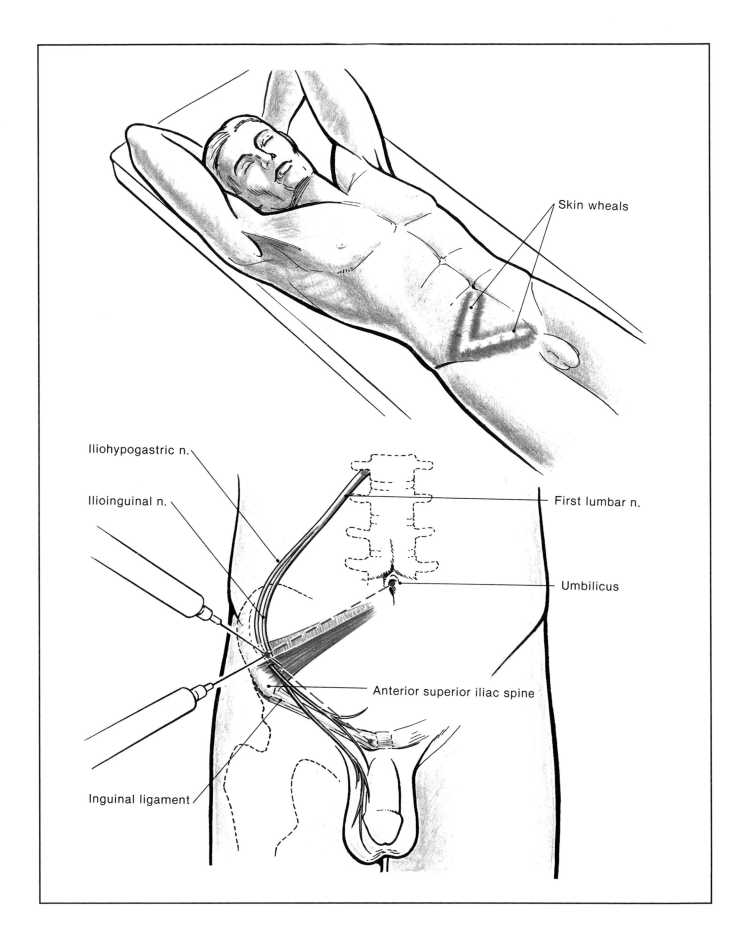

Skin wheals

Iliohypogastric n.

Ilioinguinal n.

First lumbar n.

Umbilicus

Anterior superior iliac spine

Inguinal ligament

Pelvis

Sacral Nerves

CAUDAL APPROACH—SINGLE-INJECTION TECHNIQUE

Anatomy

The sacrum, a triangular-shaped bone, is the result of fusion of the five sacral vertebrae. The upper border articulates with the fifth lumbar vertebra; the inferior edge likewise with the coccyx.

The posterior surface of the sacrum has a middle ridge, similar to the dorsal spines in the lumbar and thoracic regions. The extent of this ridge varies, usually from S1 to S3 or S4. Ordinarily there is a defect in the midline where the fifth sacral laminae would have met. There are many variations, however, and any presentation, including a complete lack of fusion, can occur. Usually the lack of fusion of the fifth sacral arch leads to an opening between the sacrum and the coccyx called the sacral hiatus. This hiatus is covered by the sacrococcygeal ligament. Lateral to and on both sides of the midline crest are four posterior sacral foramina.

The ventral surface of the sacrum, which is tilted forward at its terminal end, has four corresponding anterior sacral foramina through which the anterior primary divisions of the sacral nerves leave.

Of importance in performing a caudal nerve block is the anatomy of the sacral hiatus and sacral canal. The sacral hiatus is a triangular-shaped opening that exists because of the lack of fusion of the fifth sacral laminae. Its inferior edge is the upper border of the coccyx. Laterally, the unfused ends of the fifth sacral laminae, called the sacral cornu, are the dominant bony features.

The sacral canal is defined as the space from above the sacral hiatus to the end of the dura, at about the level of S1. Its anterior boundary is the body of the sacrum. The posterior wall is the fused dorsal laminae of S1 through S4. The superior border is the end of the dura and the inferior edge is the sacrococcygeal ligament. Within the canal are the sacral nerves, fatty tissue, and blood vessels. The size of the sacral canal varies tremendously, with volumes documented ranging from 15 to 60 cc.

The description above is of common sacrum presentations. It must be noted that multiple bony anomalies occur. These can affect more than just the shape of the bone itself. Wide discrepancies in the pattern of dorsal fusion can affect the size and position of the sacral hiatus, the size and number of dorsal sacral foramina, presence or absence of a midline sacral ridge, and so on. Peculiarities must be noted and considered before attempting caudal or transsacral nerve block.

Technique

The patient is positioned prone with a small pillow beneath the pelvis. The table is flexed at the level of the hips. The patient is asked to abduct the legs, toes turned inward. The sacral hiatus is identified by palpating the dorsal spine of the lower lumbar vertebra and continuing down the midline of the sacrum over the sacral ridge until the hiatus is encountered. The palpating finger should now rest on the opening to the caudal canal and between the sacral cornu, which are the nonfused dorsal laminae of the fifth sacral arch. This position of the coccyx can be confirmed with ballottement from below. This tenses the sacrococcygeal ligament.

A skin wheal is raised in the midline, slightly above an imaginary line between the two sacral cornu. A ¾-inch, 23-gauge needle (in the thin patient; may range to a 1 ½-inch, 22-gauge needle in the heavier patient) is advanced directly toward the hiatus at a very slight angle. Because of the increased pelvic tilt, the angle is steeper for the female patient. The needle will be felt to pierce the sacrococcygeal ligament. The ligament offers moderate resistance and once it is pierced the operator feels as if the needle has advanced into an empty space.

A test dose of 4 cc of local anesthetic with epinephrine 1 : 200,000 should be injected after negative aspiration to ensure that the tip is neither intravascular nor subarachnoid. Depending on the size of the patient and the extent of analgesia required, a volume of 15 to 20 cc of local anesthetic is injected.

Note: The piercing of the sacrococcygeal ligament is a distinct end point. The injection of the local anesthetic should be accomplished without feeling any resistance. If resistance is encountered the needle either lies in soft tissue superficial to the caudal canal or is subperiosteal; in both cases it must be repositioned.

Note: In the individual whose landmarks are difficult to palpate after the needle is thought to have passed through the sacrococcygeal ligament, 3 cc of sterile saline can be injected rapidly through the needle while the fingers of the other hand palpate over where the needle tip is presumed to be. When the needle is in the caudal canal there will be no sensation felt by the palpating fingers and the fluid should inject easily. If the needle tip is in the subcutaneous tissue, extravasation will be felt; if the needle is subperiosteal, injection will be very difficult.

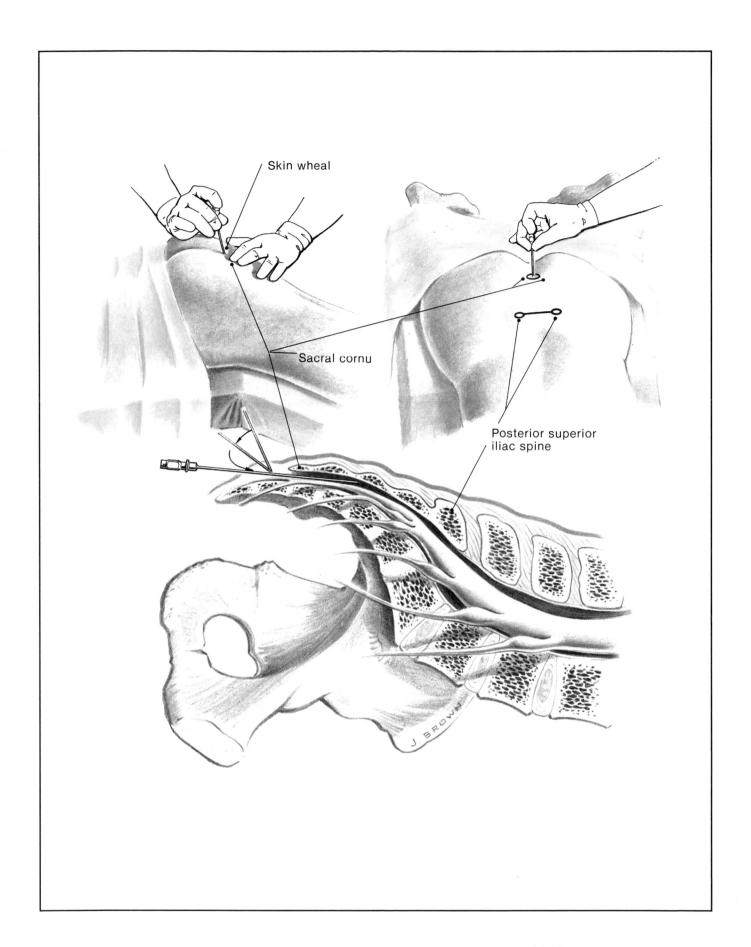

Skin wheal

Sacral cornu

Posterior superior
iliac spine

J BROWN

Sacral Nerves

CAUDAL APPROACH—CONTINUOUS TECHNIQUE

Anatomy

See anatomy for Sacral Nerves—Caudal Approach, Single-Injection Technique (p. 124).

Technique

The patient is positioned and the sacral hiatus identified as described for the caudal nerve block—single injection (p. 124). After infiltrating the skin and subcutaneous tissue with small amounts of local anesthetic, a 17- or 18-gauge, 2- to 3-inch, thin-wall needle should be advanced through the sacrococcygeal ligament. When this ligament is pierced a distinct give or popping sensation is felt. The needle is then advanced an additional ½ inch into the caudal canal and an appropriate catheter is inserted 1 inch beyond the needle tip. The needle is withdrawn and the catheter is secured in place.

After careful aspiration to ensure that neither cerebrospinal fluid nor blood returns, a test dose of 4 cc of local anesthetic with epinephrine 1:200,000 is injected and the procedure continues as noted on page 124.

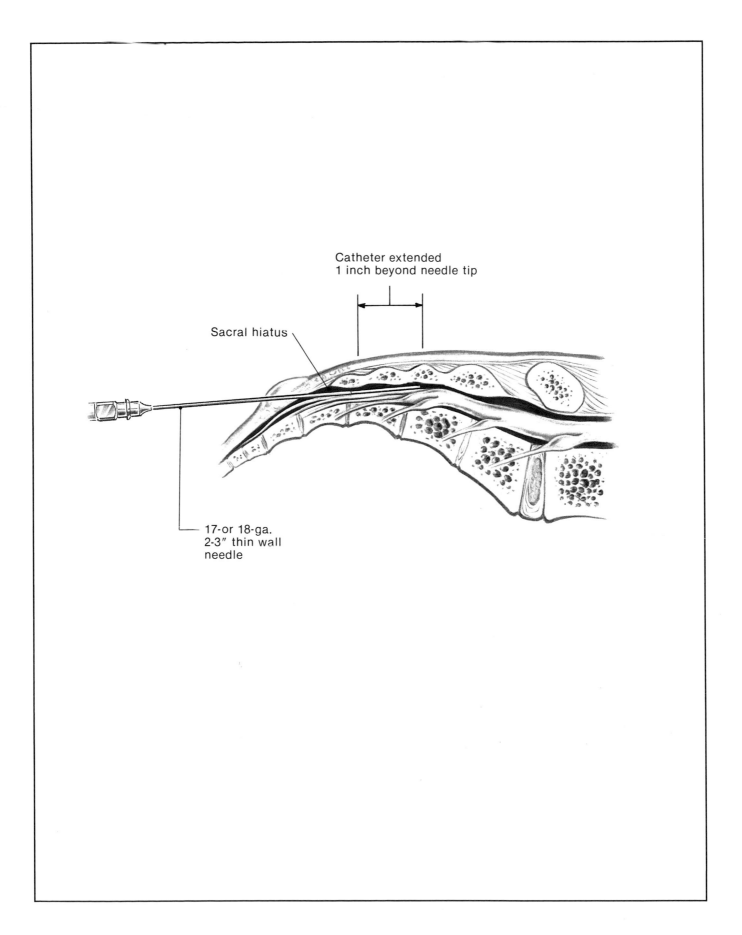

Catheter extended
1 inch beyond needle tip

Sacral hiatus

17-or 18-ga.
2-3″ thin wall
needle

Sacral Nerves

TRANSSACRAL APPROACH

Anatomy

There are usually four posterior sacral foramina that lie on a line going from 1 inch medial to and above the posterior superior iliac spine to ½ inch lateral and superior to the sacral cornu. The foramina are about ½ inch in diameter and are separated by approximately ½ to 1 inch, depending on the length of the sacrum. Through these openings pass the posterior primary divisions of the sacral nerves that provide innervation to the midline structures.

Technique

The patient is positioned as for a caudal anesthetic (p. 124). The posterior superior iliac spine and the sacral cornu are identified. About ½ to 1 inch medial and inferior to the posterior iliac spine lies the S2 foramen. Approximately ½ inch superior and lateral to the sacral cornu is the S4 foramen. At a point midway between these two is the S3 foramen. The S1 foramen is ½ to 1 inch above S2. In many cases these depressions in the posterior plate of the sacrum can be palpated through the skin.

A skin wheal is made just superior to the location of the S2 foramen, and through it a 2-inch, 22-gauge block needle is inserted perpendicular to the posterior plate of the sacrum. After encountering the sacrum the needle is walked down its posterior plate until the foramen is entered, then advanced ¼ to ½ inch. The procedure is similar for S1, S3, and S4. Three to five cubic centimeters of local anesthetic is injected in each location after careful aspiration.

Note: It must be remembered that the anatomy of the sacrum is quite variable. The technique presented here applies only for the usual anatomic presentation.

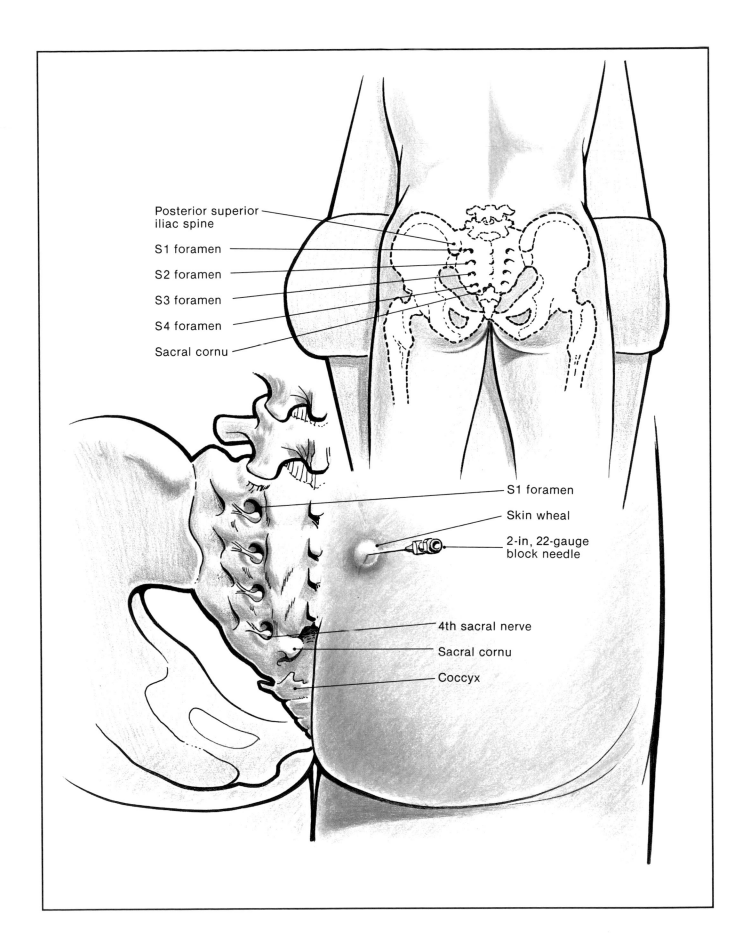

Posterior superior
iliac spine

S1 foramen

S2 foramen

S3 foramen

S4 foramen

Sacral cornu

S1 foramen

Skin wheal

2-in, 22-gauge
block needle

4th sacral nerve

Sacral cornu

Coccyx

Fifth Sacral and Coccygeal Nerves

Anatomy

The coccygeal nerve emerges from the caudal canal via the sacral hiatus. It fuses with branches of the posterior primary divisions of S4 and S5 to supply the skin over the coccyx. The fifth sacral nerve exits via the sacral hiatus and travels medial and inferior to the sacral cornu.

Technique

The patient lies in the same position as for caudal block (p. 124). The inferior edge of the fifth sacral cornu is palpated and at this point a 1-inch, 23-gauge block needle is inserted and directed toward the midline. Three cubic centimeters of local anesthetic is infiltrated as the needle advances toward the coccyx. The needle is then redirected slightly to go just medial and deep to the sacral cornu and an additional 2 cc of local anesthetic is injected. The first infiltration will block the coccygeal nerve; the second injection will block the fifth sacral nerve.

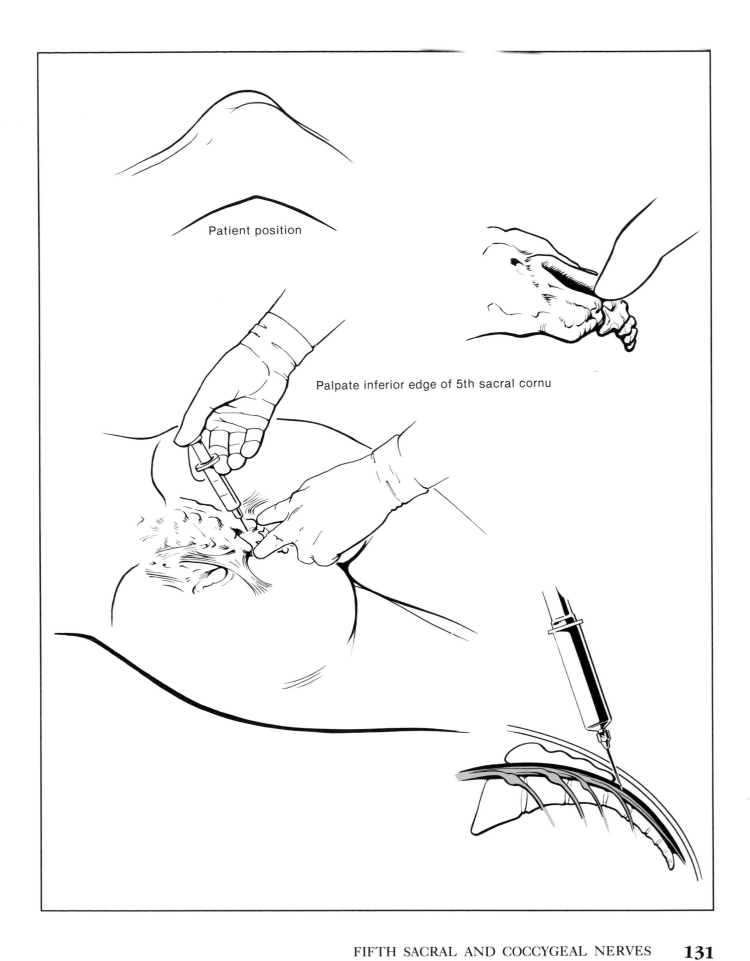

Patient position

Palpate inferior edge of 5th sacral cornu

Pudendal Nerve

TECHNIQUE 1—FOR FEMALES

Anatomy

The pudendal nerve arises from S2, S3, and S4. It leaves the pelvis in close proximity to the sciatic nerve between the piriformis and coccygeus muscles and enters the gluteal region through the inferior part of the greater sciatic notch, where it lies adjacent to the sacrospinous ligament. The nerve then passes through the lesser sciatic notch to enter the pudendal canal. There the nerve gives off the inferior rectal nerve and soon divides into its terminal divisions—the perineal and dorsal nerves of the penis (in the male) and clitoris (in the female).

Technique

The patient lies in a slightly exaggerated lithotomy position. The index and middle fingers of the operator's hand is inserted through the vagina to rest on the ischial spine. A needle guide is inserted between the fingers until its tip is against the vaginal wall just proximinal to the ischial spine. A 5-inch, 20-gauge block needle is inserted through the guide, the vaginal wall is pierced, and the needle is advanced into and through the sacrospinous ligament, going just posterior to the ischial spine. A definite loss of resistance is felt when the needle pierces the ligament. Ten cubic centimeters of local anesthetic is infiltrated at this point and an additional 5 to 10 cc is injected as the needle is withdrawn slowly toward the vagina.

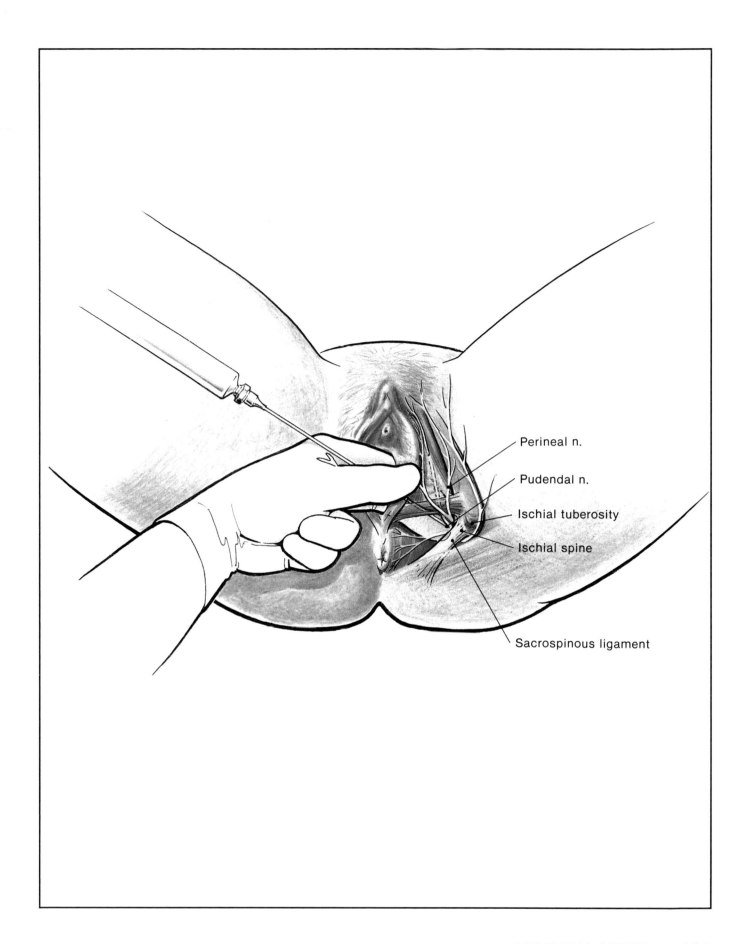

Perineal n.

Pudendal n.

Ischial tuberosity

Ischial spine

Sacrospinous ligament

Pudendal Nerve

TECHNIQUE 2—FOR MALES OR FEMALES

Anatomy

See anatomy for Pudendal Nerve, Technique 1—for Females (p. 132).

Technique

The patient is positioned as for Technique 1 (p. 132). The ischial tuberosity is identified and a skin wheal is made over its inferior and medial border. A 4- to 6-inch, 20-gauge block needle is guided through the soft tissue of the perineum to the ischial spine by an index finger placed in either the rectum or vagina. After the spine is contacted the needle is moved slightly medial and deeper to pierce the sacrococcygeal ligament as described for Technique 1. Ten cubic centimeters of local anesthetic is then injected and an additional 5 to 10 cc is infiltrated as the needle is withdrawn past the ischial spine.

Note: If only the peripheral perineal branch of the pudendal nerve has to be blocked, 5 to 10 cc of local anesthetic can be deposited in the ischiorectal fossa, the area between the ischial tuberosity and the ischial spine.

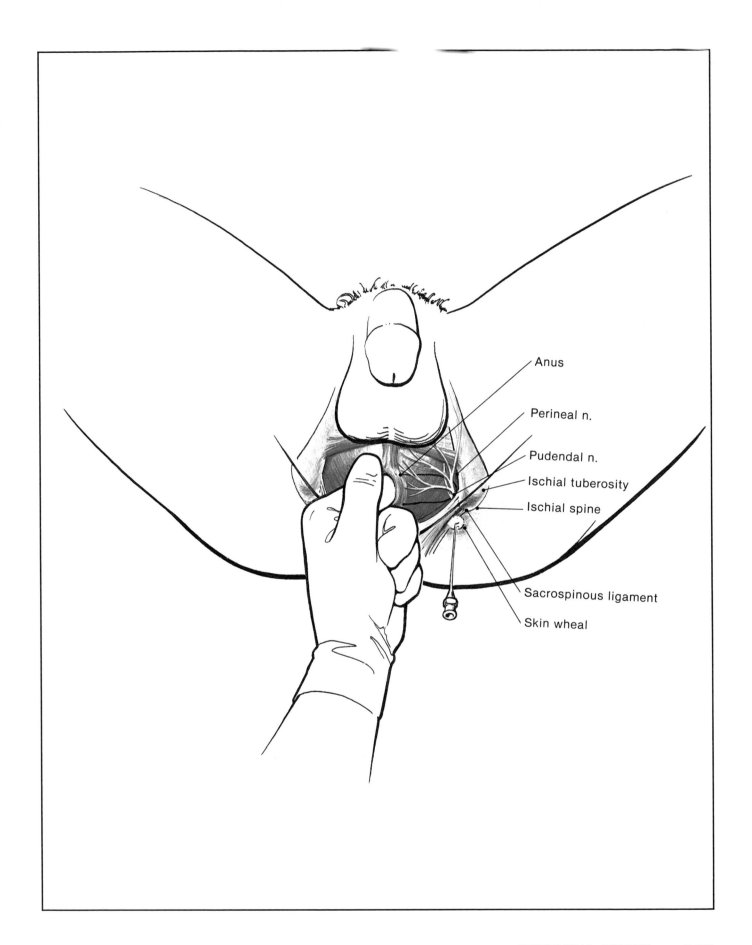

Anus

Perineal n.

Pudendal n.

Ischial tuberosity

Ischial spine

Sacrospinous ligament

Skin wheal

Paracervical Block

Anatomy

Surrounding the lower portions of the uterus and upper cervix are the inferior hypogastric (pelvic) and uterine plexuses. Sensory fibers from these ascend to the superior hypogastric plexus and enter the cord via the lower thoracic and upper lumbar sympathetic chain ganglia.

The early mild to moderate pain of the first stage of labor is transmitted primarily via T11 and T12. However, recruitment of T10 and L1 probably occurs in the later first and second stages of labor.

During the second stage of labor other pain sensitive tissues in the perineum and pelvis are also stimulated. Primary innervation of these structures is by branches from the pudendal nerve. Block of the pudendal nerve is discussed on pages 132 and 134.

Technique

Paracervical nerve block is performed using a short-beveled needle, either with a needle guide (see Technique 1 for pudendal block, p. 132) or alone. A 5-inch needle, or first a needle guide if one is to be used, is advanced to the lateral fornix on either side of the cervix using the index and middle fingers placed in the vagina as an aid. The needle pierces the vaginal musosa to a depth of ½ to ¾ inch. This puts the needle tip in the vicinity of the inferior hypogastric nerve plexus. Ten cubic centimeters of local anesthetic is deposited after careful aspiration. The procedure is then repeated on the other side in an identical manner.

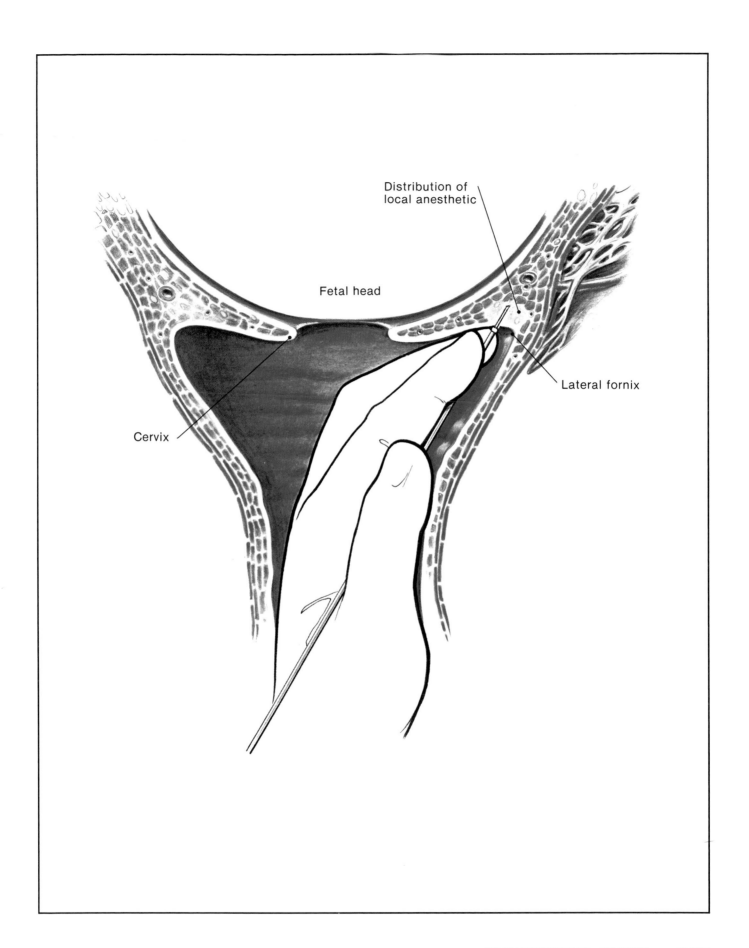

Distribution of
local anesthetic

Fetal head

Lateral fornix

Cervix

Penis

Anatomy

The dorsal nerve, a branch of the pudendal nerve, is the major innervation of the penis. The dorsal nerve divides at the base of the penis into a major anterior division and minor posterior branches. These smaller branches supply the underside of the penis and frenulum while the larger branch supplies the remainder of the organ. The skin around the base of the penis also gets contributions from the genitofemoral and ilioinguinal nerves.

Technique

A triangle of local anesthetic is placed at the base of the penis, with the pubic tubercles and a point just inferior to the undersurface of the penis on the scrotum as the corners of the triangle. This is accomplished with about 10 to 15 cc of local anesthetic using a 2- to 3-inch, 22-gauge block needle.

The area surrounding the dorsal nerve of the penis is then infiltrated by piercing the fascia (Buck's fascia) with a 25-gauge needle at about the 10:30 and 1:30 positions and injecting 1 cc of local anesthetic at each site. This should be done close to the base of the penis, before the dorsal nerve divides. If it is not possible to block the nerve prior to division, it is necessary to separately anesthetize the ventral branches. This is accomplished by infiltrating 1 cc of local anesthetic between the corpora cavernosa and the corpus spongiosum on the ventral side of the penis.

For procedures on the tip of the penis such as circumcision, only injection of the dorsal nerves and infiltration of the frenulum is necessary.

Note: Local anesthetics used for all blocks of the penis should not contain epinephrine or any other vasoconstrictor.

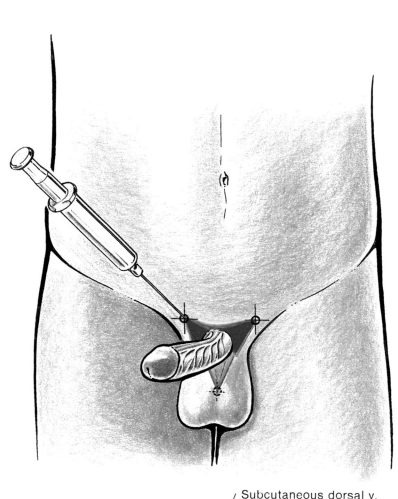

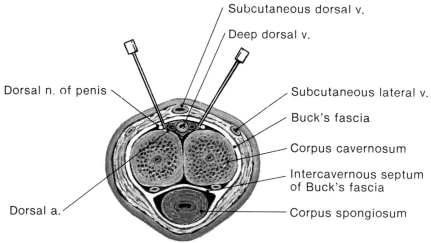

Subcutaneous dorsal v.

Deep dorsal v.

Dorsal n. of penis

Subcutaneous lateral v.

Buck's fascia

Corpus cavernosum

Intercavernous septum
of Buck's fascia

Dorsal a.

Corpus spongiosum

Rectum and Anus

Anatomy

The perianal skin and anal sphincter receive their nerve supply from branches of the sacral plexus, primarily S2, S3, and S4. Terminal fibers from S5 and the coccygeal nerve may provide additional sensory innervation.

Technique

With the patient in the lithotomy or prone position skin wheals are raised at 12, 3, 6, and 9 o'clock at the level where the anal mucosa comes in contact with the skin. The skin wheals are connected by a subcutaneous ring of local anesthesic using a 1½-inch, 23-gauge needle. Through each skin wheal 5 cc of local anesthetic is injected using a fresh needle, thus infiltrating the soft tissue surrounding the mucosa of the rectum and the rectal sphincter. A finger should be in the rectum to ascertain that the needle tip does not pierce the mucosa. Adequate surface anesthesia as well as relaxation of the rectal sphincter will be produced.

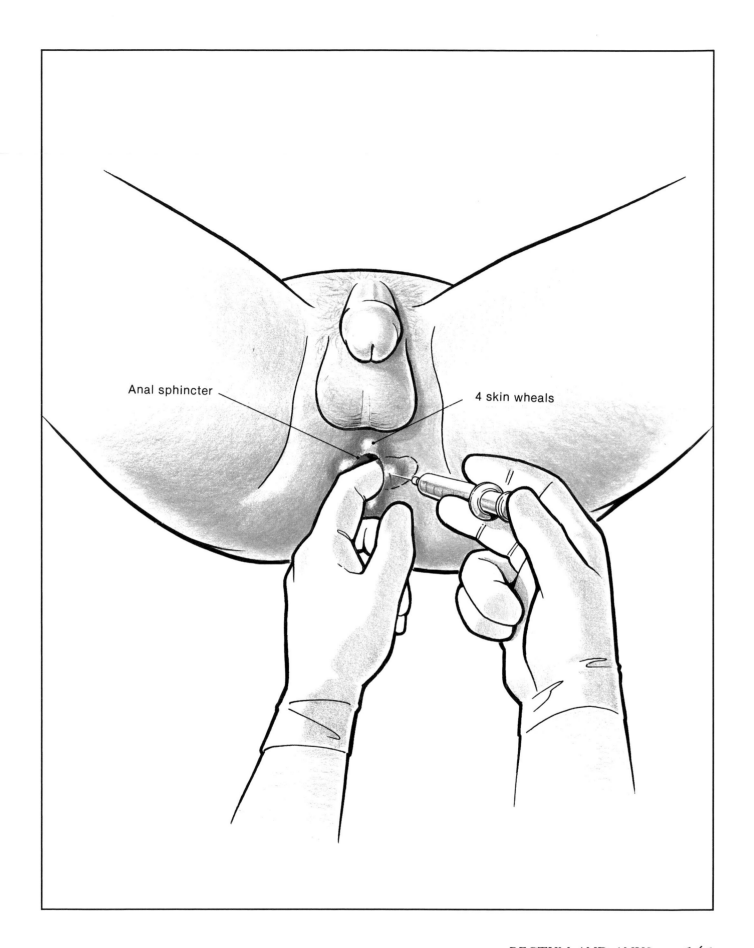

Anal sphincter

4 skin wheals

Lower Extremity

Sciatic Nerve

POSTERIOR APPROACH

Anatomy

The sciatic nerve, largest nerve in the body, originates from the anterior divisions of L4 and L5, S1, S2, and S3. The roots fuse and leave the pelvis through the greater sciatic notch below the piriform muscle. The sciatic nerve lies approximately midway between the ischial tuberosity and greater trochanter of the femur, below the lower part of the gluteus maximus muscle. In the thigh the nerve gives off branches to the hamstring muscles and adductor magnus muscle. About one-half or two-thirds of the way down the thigh the nerve splits into its two major components, the tibial and common peroneal nerves.

Technique

With the patient in Sim's position, the superior border of the greater trochanter and the posterior superior iliac spine are palpated. Midway on a line between these points and at a right angle approximately 2 inches inferior a skin wheal is raised. A 3- to 4-inch, 22-gauge block needle, depending on the size of the patient, is inserted perpendicular to the skin and passed through the soft tissue until a paresthesia going to the lower leg or foot is obtained. This usually occurs at a depth of from 2 to 3½ inches. If the bone of the sciatic notch is contacted first, the needle should be withdrawn and the point directed slightly cephalad along the perpendicular line drawn previously. If a paresthesia is still not obtained, provided the periosteum is continually met, the needle should be reinserted slightly lateral and the procedure repeated. Ten to fifteen cubic centimeters of a concentrated local anesthetic solution is required.

Note: Obtaining a paresthesia is almost mandatory for the block to be adequate.

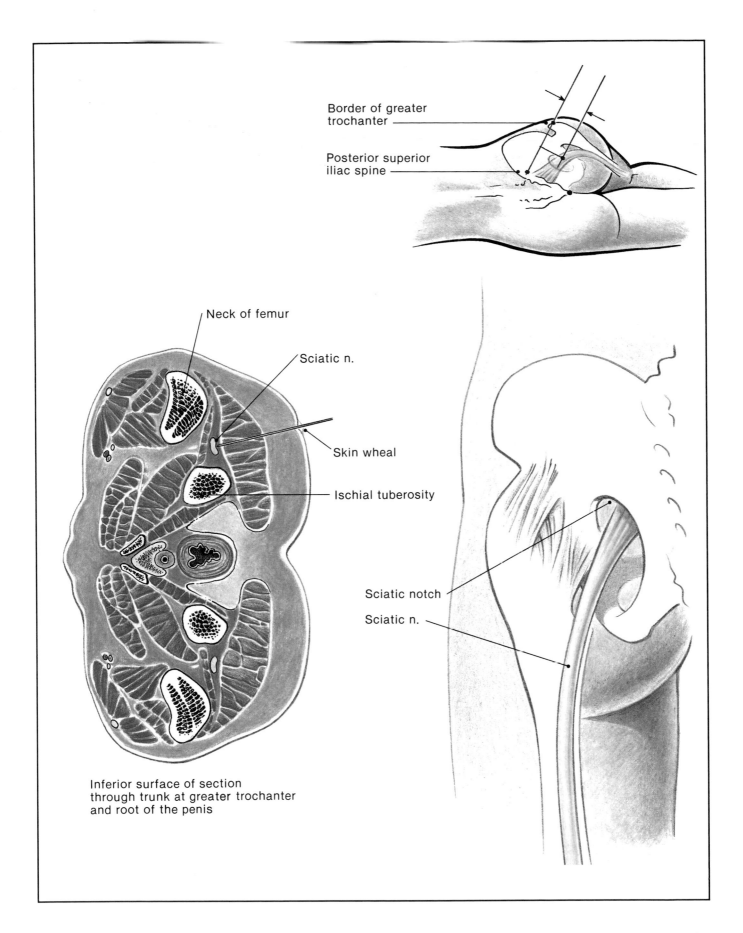

Border of greater trochanter

Posterior superior iliac spine

Neck of femur

Sciatic n.

Skin wheal

Ischial tuberosity

Sciatic notch

Sciatic n.

Inferior surface of section through trunk at greater trochanter and root of the penis

Sciatic Nerve

LITHOTOMY APPROACH

Anatomy

See anatomy for Sciatic Nerve—Posterior Approach (p. 144).

Technique

The patient lies supine with the leg flexed to more than a 90 degree angle at the hip level, maintained in this position by an assistant. Just above the gluteal fold and in the middle of the thigh a skin wheal is made. A 3-inch, 22-gauge block needle is inserted perpendicular to the skin in the general direction of the femur. A paresthesia is usually obtained as the needle is advanced to a depth of 2 to 2½ inches. If a paresthesia is not obtained the needle should be moved fanwise from medial to lateral until one is elicited. Ten to fifteen cubic centimeters of a concentrated local anesthetic solution is then deposited.

Note: A definite paresthesia to the lower leg or foot is required for a successful block.

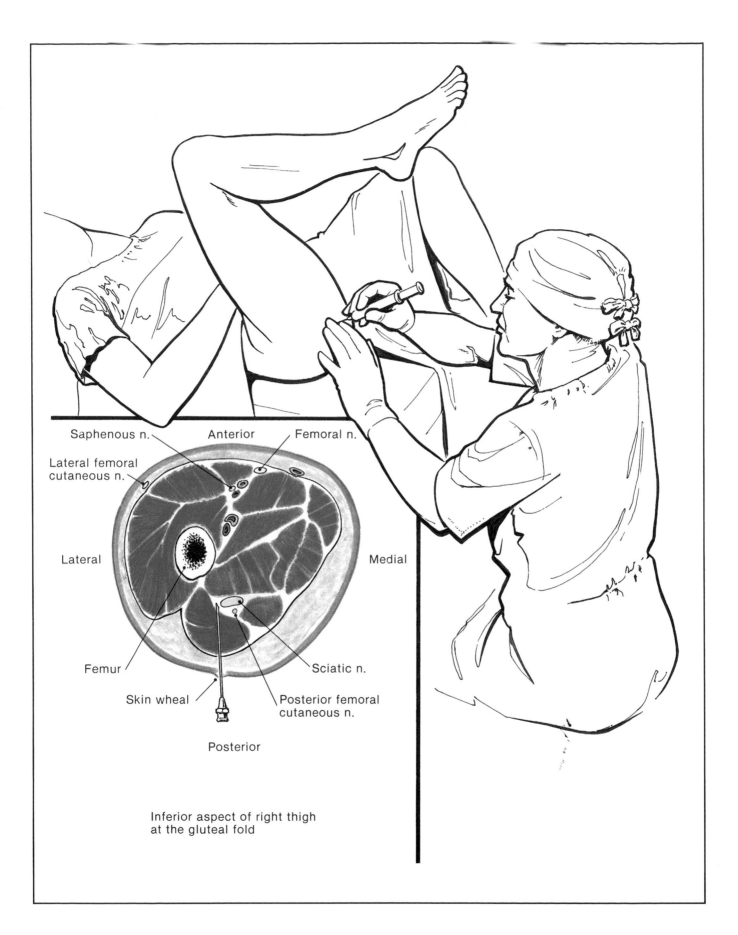

Saphenous n.　　Anterior　　Femoral n.

Lateral femoral
cutaneous n.

Lateral　　　　　　　　　　　　　　　　　Medial

Femur

Skin wheal

Sciatic n.

Posterior femoral
cutaneous n.

Posterior

Inferior aspect of right thigh
at the gluteal fold

Femoral Nerve

Anatomy

The femoral nerve arises from the fusion in the psoas muscle of the dorsal divisions of the anterior rami of the second, third, and fourth lumbar segments. It exits the muscle laterally, entering the iliac fossa and providing motor fibers to the iliac muscle. It then passes into the thigh underneath the inguinal ligament and just lateral to femoral artery. The acronym NAVEL describes the lateral to medial positions of the structures of the neurovascular bundle just below the level of the inguinal ligament in the femoral sheath—Nerve, Artery, Vein, Empty space, and Lymphatics.

The femoral nerve sends muscle fibers to the sartorius, quadriceps femoris, and pectineus muscles. Sensory branches go to the skin overlying the anterior and lower medial portions of the thigh. It continues down into the lower leg as the saphenous nerve.

Technique

The patient lies supine. The femoral artery is identified as it emerges into the leg under the inguinal ligament. Just lateral to the palpating finger and as close to the inguinal ligament as possible a ½- to 1-inch, 22-gauge block needle is inserted through a skin wheal. Paresthesias are sought as the needle pierces the subcutaneous fat. If one is not obtained, needle is moved fanwise from medial to lateral and 15 cc of local anesthetic is injected. If a paresthesia has been obtained, 8 to 10 cc of local anesthetic solution will provide an adequate block.

Note: If the patient has an extremely large thigh, a longer needle may be required.

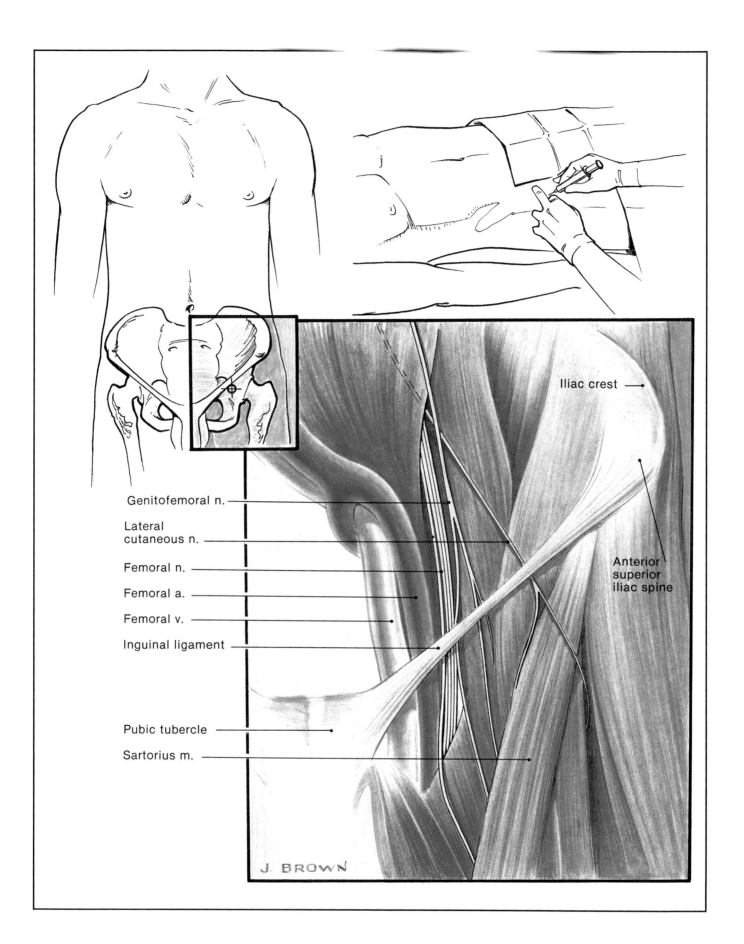

Iliac crest

Genitofemoral n.

Lateral
cutaneous n.

Femoral n.

Femoral a.

Femoral v.

Inguinal ligament

Anterior
superior
iliac spine

Pubic tubercle

Sartorius m.

J. BROWN

Lateral Femoral Cutaneous Nerve

Anatomy

The lateral femoral cutaneous nerve is formed from the posterior divisions of L2 and L3 within the substance of the psoas muscle. It passes laterally just beneath the rim of the pelvis to enter the thigh close to the anterior superior iliac spine behind the inguinal ligament. After piercing the fascia, sensory branches are distributed to the lateral buttock and thigh, occasionally as far as the knee joint.

Technique

The patient lies supine. The anterior superior iliac spine is palpated, as is the inguinal ligament. At a point approximately ½ to 1 inch medial to the anterior superior iliac spine and just inferior to the inguinal ligament a 2-inch, 22-gauge block needle is inserted perpendicular to the skin. When the needle has passed beneath the fascia a paresthesia may be elicited. The exact needle depth depends on the amount of soft tissue, but usually it is from ½ to 1 ½ inches. If the bone is contacted prior to obtaining a paresthesia, the needle is withdrawn to the subcutaneous tissue and the same process repeated in fanwise directions. Once a paresthesia is elicited, 5 to 8 cc of solution is injected. Occasionally when no paresthesia can be obtained local anesthetic is spread beneath the fascia.

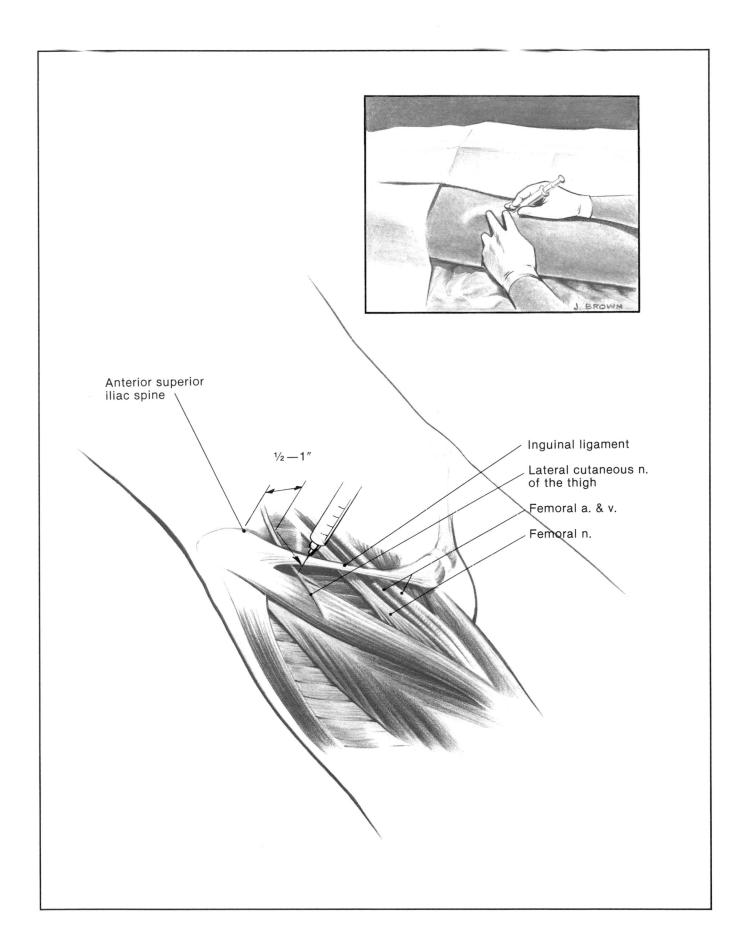

Anterior superior
iliac spine

½ — 1″

Inguinal ligament

Lateral cutaneous n.
of the thigh

Femoral a. & v.

Femoral n.

J. BROWN

Obturator Nerve

Anatomy

The obturator nerve originates from the ventral branches of L2, L3, and L4, which form a common trunk in the substance of the psoas muscle. It emerges from the medial border of this muscle to enter the pelvis. The nerve passes downward with the obturator vessels and leaves the pelvis through the obturator canal to enter the thigh. It terminates by giving sensory innervation to most of the medial portion of the thigh. In its course, branches are given off to the hip joint, the external obturator, gracilis, and adductor muscles. The posterior division of the nerve supplies an articular branch to the knee joint.

Technique

The patient lies supine with legs slightly spread. The spine of the pubic bone on the involved side is identified and a skin wheal is made 1 inch lateral and inferior to it. After generous infiltration with local anesthetic, a 3-inch block needle is inserted perpendicular to the skin wheal until the upper part of the inferior ramus of the pubic bone is contacted. This should be at a depth of ½ to 1 inch. The needle is redirected to slip past the inferior ramus and just underneath the superior ramus of the pubic bone, then advanced an additional 1 ½ inch. This needle direction is lateral and slightly inferior. The needle tip should now lie in the area of the obturator foramen. Paresthesias are only occasionally elicited. Ten to fifteen cubic centimeters of local anesthesia is infiltrated as the needle is moved back and forth slowly.

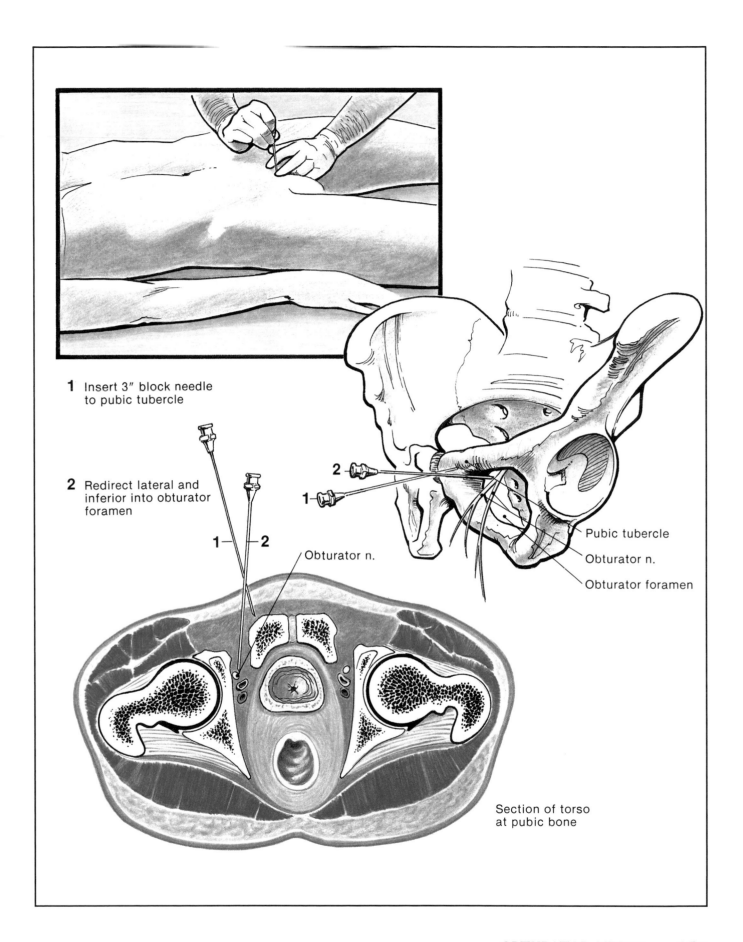

1 Insert 3″ block needle to pubic tubercle

2 Redirect lateral and inferior into obturator foramen

1 — 2

Obturator n.

2

1

Pubic tubercle

Obturator n.

Obturator foramen

Section of torso at pubic bone

OBTURATOR NERVE   **153**

Common Peroneal Nerve

Anatomy

The common peroneal nerve arises from the fourth and fifth lumbar and first and second sacral trunks. Along with the tibial nerve, it is one of the two major peripheral continuations of the sciatic nerve. It moves laterally from its origin at the bifurcation of the sciatic to enter the leg behind the head of the fibula. It then winds laterally on the neck of the fibula to enter the upper part of the peroneus longus muscle, where it divides into its terminal branches—the deep peroneal and superficial peroneal nerves.

In its course the common peroneal nerve gives off various muscular branches, a twig to the knee joint, and, via its lateral cutaneous branch, sensory supply to the skin of the back and lateral side of the upper portion of the calf.

Technique

With the patient lying in the lateral position, the head and neck of the fibula are palpated. Many times the common peroneal nerve can be felt in the subcutaneous tissue at the junction of the head and neck of the fibula. A 1 ½-inch, 23-gauge block needle is inserted through a skin wheal in the direction of the bone and 5 cc of local anesthetic is infiltrated as the needle advances from the subcutaneous area to the neck of the fibula. Often a paresthesia will occur. If so, the remaining local anesthetic should be deposited at that point.

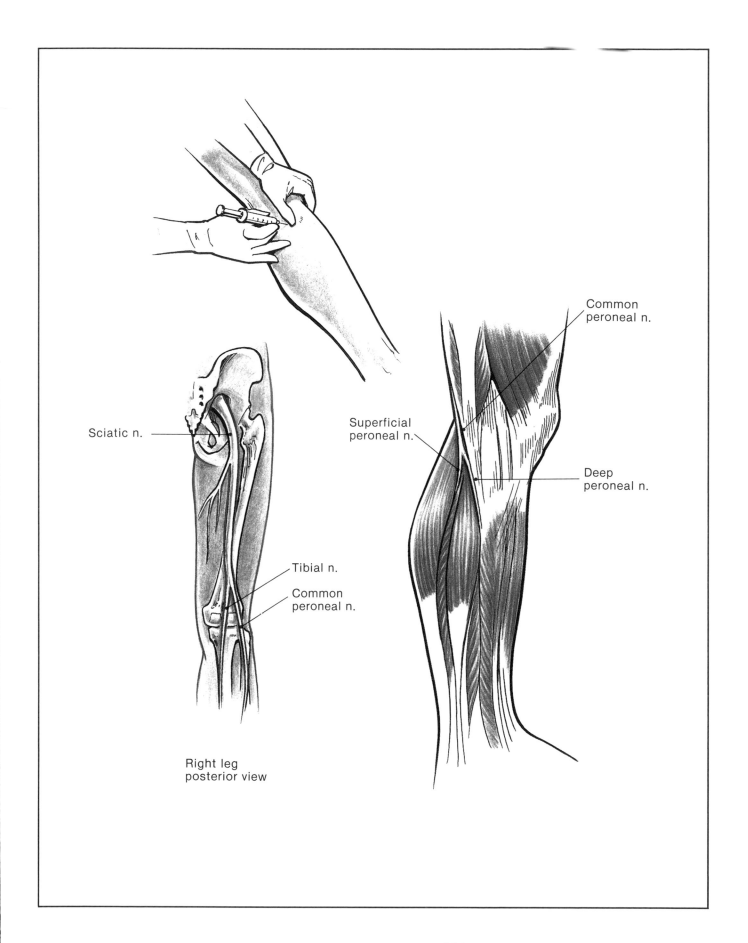

Sciatic n.

Tibial n.

Common
peroneal n.

Right leg
posterior view

Common
peroneal n.

Superficial
peroneal n.

Deep
peroneal n.

Saphenous Nerve

Anatomy

The saphenous nerve is the largest sensory branch of the femoral nerve, deriving its fibers from L3 and L4. It descends in the thigh lateral to the femoral artery, becoming subcutaneous behind the medial femoral condyle. The nerve supplies the skin over the medial side of the leg and ankle and a variable distance onto the foot.

Technique

The patient lies in the lateral position and the medial condyle of the femur is identified. The saphenous nerve can often be palpated here. If not, a skin wheal is raised and a 1½-inch, 23-gauge block needle is slowly advanced, infiltrating local anesthetic until the femur is encountered. Additional local anesthetic should be injected as the needle is withdrawn. A total of 5 to 7 cc may be required.

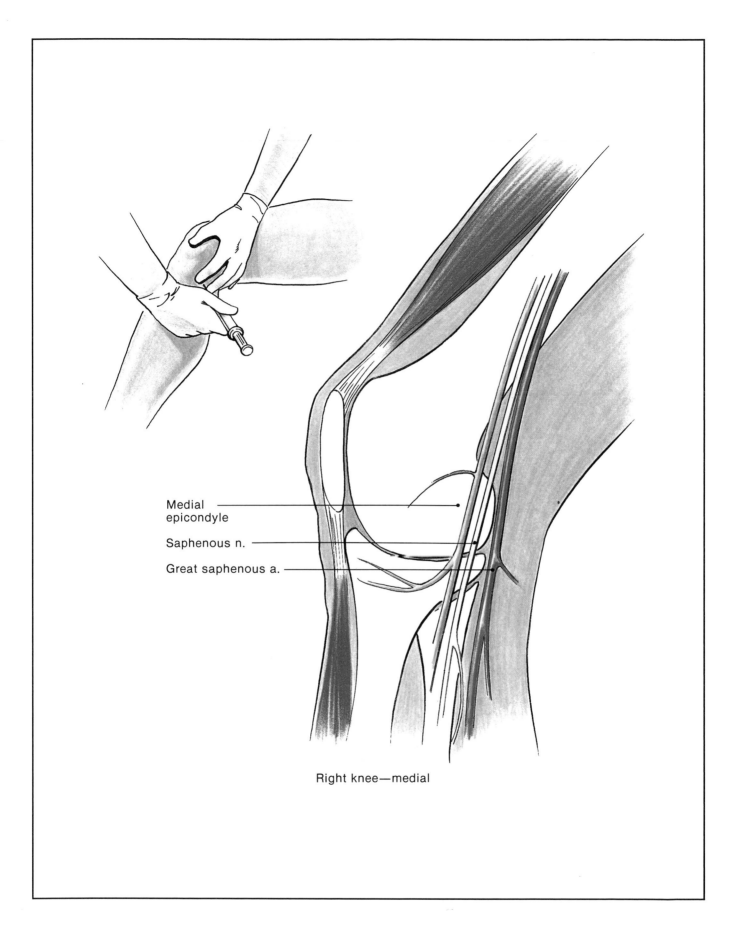

Medial
epicondyle

Saphenous n.

Great saphenous a.

Right knee—medial

Deep Peroneal Nerve

Anatomy

The deep peroneal nerve is the continuation of the common peroneal nerve that arises in the upper leg. It runs down the leg in the anterior compartment with the tibial vessels to the ankle joint, where it divides into terminal branches. The nerve enters the foot just medial to the tendon of the hallucis longus muscle. It supplies fibers to several extensor muscles, the tarsal and metatarsal joints, and the skin of the opposing halves of the first and second toes.

Technique

The patient lies supine and the tendon of the hallucis longus muscle is palpated during extension of the big toe against resistance. A 1½-inch, 23-gauge block needle is inserted just medial to the tendon and perpendicular to the tibia. As the needle is advanced toward the tibia a paresthesia involving the distribution of the deep peroneal nerve may be encountered, noted as a tingling sensation going into the toes. If the paresthesia is not elicited, the needle is advanced until the tibia is contacted and 5 to 8 cc of local anesthetic deposited as the needle is slowly withdrawn toward the skin.

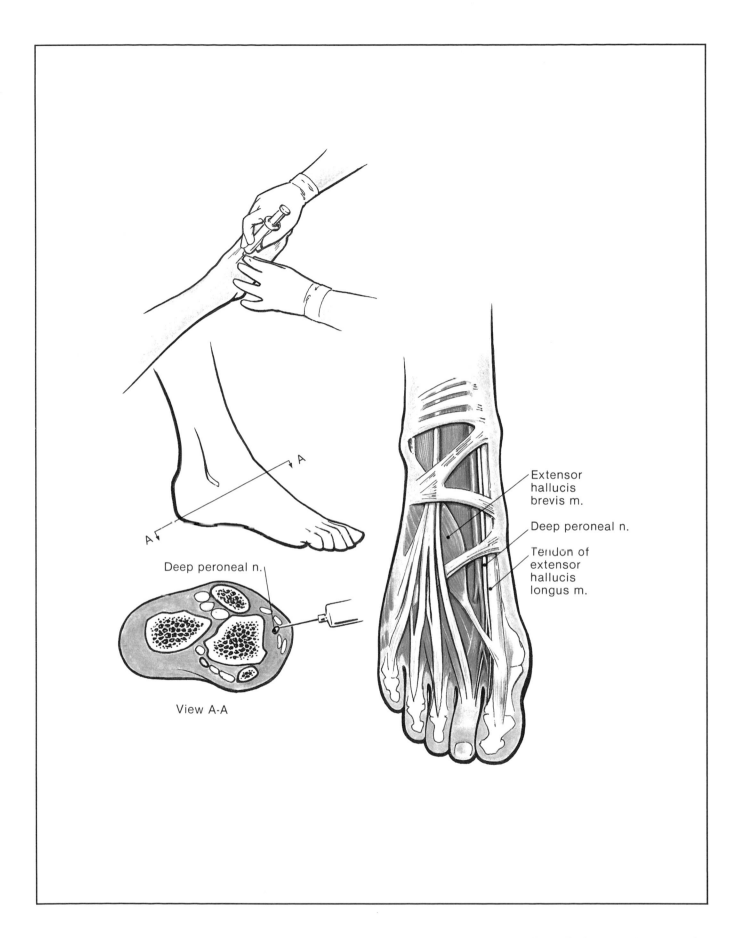

Extensor
hallucis
brevis m.

Deep peroneal n.

Tendon of
extensor
hallucis
longus m.

Deep peroneal n.

View A-A

Superficial Peroneal and Saphenous Nerves

Anatomy

The superficial peroneal nerve is a branch of the common peroneal nerve. It descends the leg adjacent to the extensor digitorum longus muscle where it divides into terminal branches just above the ankle. Its terminal fibers supply sensation to the dorsum of the foot and the adjacent sides of the first through fifth toes.

The anatomy of the saphenous nerve has been described on page 156. Its terminal branches enter the foot between the edge of the extensor hallucis longus tendon and the medial malleolus.

Technique

The saphenous nerve is blocked by running a subcutaneous wheal of local anesthetic from the site of needle insertion for block of the deep peroneal nerve medially to the anterior surface of the medial malleolus. The superficial peroneal nerve is blocked by running a subcutaneous wheal of local anesthetic laterally from the site of insertion of the needle for the deep peroneal nerve to the anterior surface of the lateral malleolus.

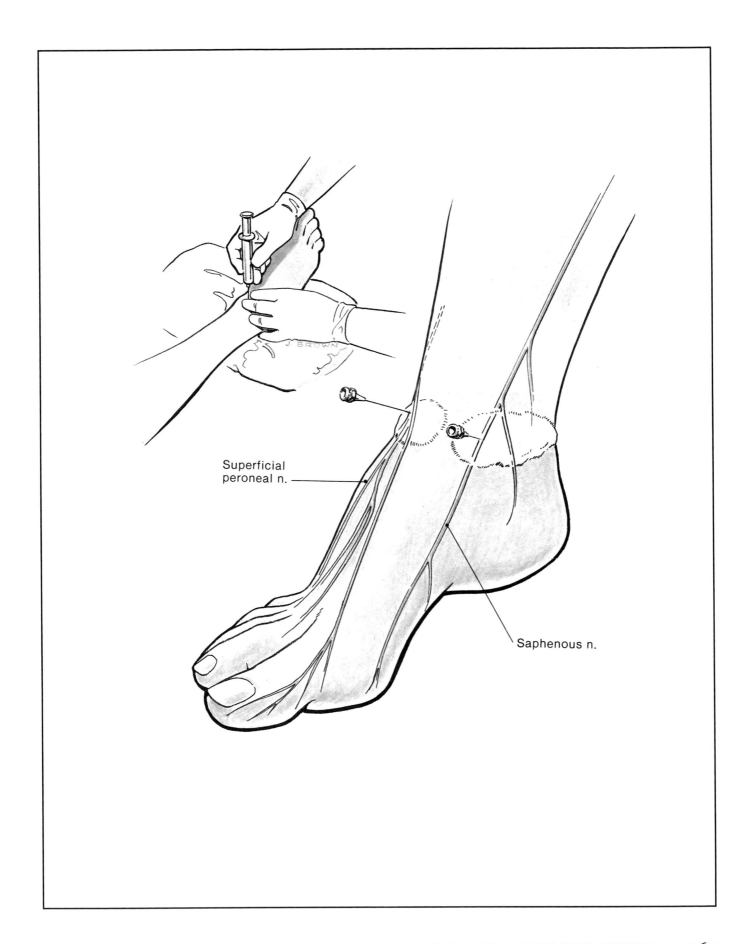

Superficial
peroneal n.

Saphenous n.

Tibial Nerve

Anatomy

The tibial nerve is the largest division of the sciatic trunk and consists of fibers from L4 to S3. It descends through the back of the calf deep to the soleus muscle. The nerve then moves medially, going between the achilles tendon and medial malleolus and dividing into the lateral and medial plantar nerves. In addition to many muscular branches, it supplies sensation to the skin of the heel and the medial side of the sole of the foot.

Technique

The foot is positioned so that the area between the medial malleolus and the achilles tendon is easily accessible. This is best done with the patient either in prone or lateral position. The posterior tibial artery is palpated (if possible) and a 1½-inch, 23-gauge block needle is directed toward the artery as it courses in the posterior groove of the medial malleolus. A paresthesia should occur before the bone is contacted. Occasionally the needle has to be fanned in a mediolateral direction until the nerve is stimulated.

If for some reason a paresthesia is not obtained, the needle is advanced until the bone is met, then withdrawn approximately ¼ to ½ inch. Five cubic centimeters of local anesthetic is injected.

Note: The terminal branches (medial and lateral plantar nerves) are also blocked with this technique.

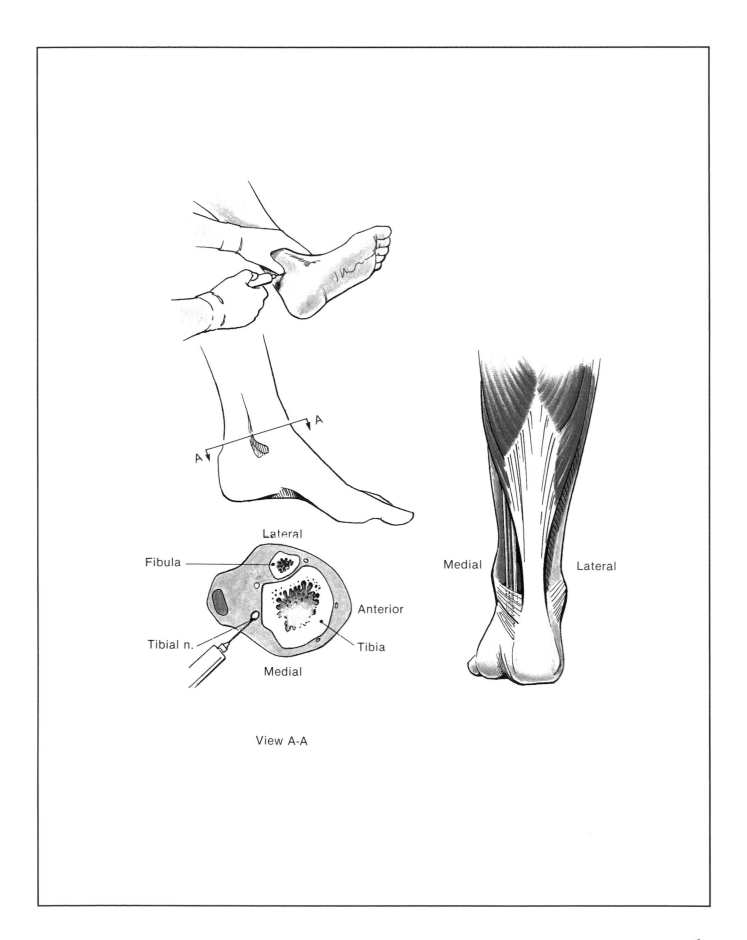

Lateral

Fibula

Anterior

Tibial n.

Tibia

Medial

View A-A

Medial

Lateral

Sural Nerve

Anatomy

The sural nerve branches from the posterior tibial nerve and descends in the posterior compartment of the leg. It enters the foot behind the lateral malleolus, between it and the achilles tendon. The nerve provides sensation to the posterior lateral aspect of the lower calf as well as the lateral side of the foot and the fifth toe.

Technique

Patient position is the same as for block of the tibial nerve. The sural nerve lies in the groove behind the lateral malleolus at approximately the same depth as the tibial nerve. A block needle is inserted just lateral to the achilles tendon aiming toward the posterior sur-face of the lateral malleolus. A paresthesia may be elicited prior to striking the bone. If not, the bone is contacted and 5 to 7 cc of local anesthetic is infiltrated as the needle is slowly withdrawn.

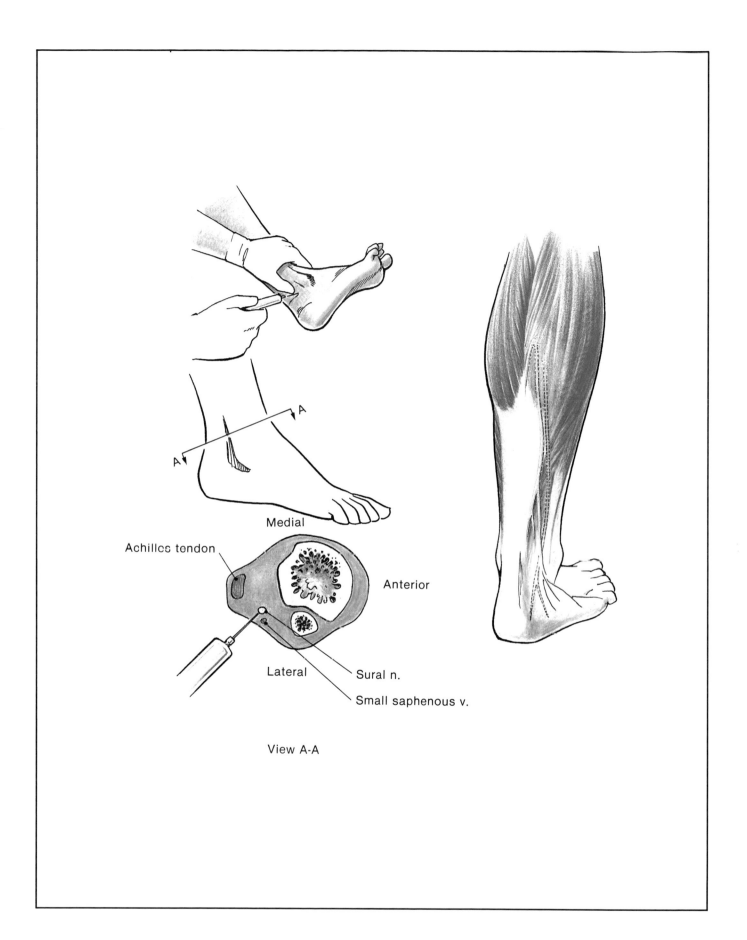

Medial

Achilles tendon

Anterior

Lateral

Sural n.

Small saphenous v.

View A-A

Spinal and Epidural

Spinal and Epidural Anatomy

The Vertebral Column

The bony spinal column consists of 24 individual vertebrae (7 cervical, 12 thoracic, 5 lumbar), the sacrum, comprised of 5 sacral vertebrae that are fused early in life, and the coccyx, which is the fusion of 4 coccygeal segments. A typical vertebra consists of the body (anterior part) and the vertebral arch (posterior part), attached to the body via the pedicles. At the junction of the pedicles and the vertebral arch, or laminae, are the transverse processes. The dorsal extension of the fused laminae is the spinous process.

The spinous processes (dorsal spines) in the lumbar area tend to be broad and somewhat shorter than the spines found in the midthoracic region. The relative position of the spines in the thoracic and lumbar areas also varies. The first and second thoracic spinous processes and the second, third, fourth, and fifth lumbar spines lie immediately above their respective vertebral bodies. From T3 to L1 the spinous processes are angulated to some degree, most prominently in the T4 to T9 area. For example, the spine of T3 overlies the T4 vertebral body. The T6 spine is even more angulated and its caudad tip may ride over the space between the T7 and T8 vertebrae.

The Ligaments of the Vertebral Column

The anterior and posterior longitudinal ligaments provide support for the bodies of the vertebrae from C2 to the upper portion of the sacrum. Between the vertebrae themselves are the intervertebral discs, each composed of a peripheral portion, the annulus fibrosis, and a central section called the nucleus pulposus. The discs are thinnest in the T3 to T7 area and thickest between the lumbar vertebrae. In both the cervical and lumbar regions the discs are thicker anteriorly than posteriorly, which contributes somewhat to the anterior convexities of the spine in these areas.

Ligaments that exist between the dorsal spines are of special significance since they need to be identified if one is going to attempt epidural or spinal nerve block. The supraspinous ligament is a tough fibrous structure that extends from the seventh cervical vertebra to the sacrum. In the lower part of the spinal column the ligament becomes both wider and stronger. The interspinous ligament connects the spinous processes of adjacent vertebrae. Its most superficial edge is in contact with the supraspinous ligament; the deeper portion comes in contact with the ligamentum flavum. The interspinous ligament is also thickest and strongest in the lumbar region.

The ligamentum flavum consists of strong elastic tissue attached to the anterior inferior surface of the laminae above and the posterior superior surface of the laminae below. The ligaments extend from the articular processes laterally to the midline. Like the supraspinous and interspinous ligaments, the ligamentum flavum is thickest in the lumbar region.

The Extradural and Intradural Spaces

The spinal dura mater is continuous with the inner meningeal layer of the intracranial dura. It starts at the foramen magnum and continues as a sac surrounding the spinal cord and its neural contents to the middle of the body of the second sacral vertebra, in the average adult patient. This terminal portion is quite variable; between 40 and 50 percent of patients have a still further caudad extension. At its termination the dura mater invests the filum terminale, which is connected to the periosteal surface of the coccyx.

Although the dura mater and arachnoid act as a single protective sheath for the spinal cord, in reality a potential space does exist between the two of them. There is a minute amount of liquid lubricating the lining between the dura and the arachnoid. It is possible to make a subdural extra-arachnoid injection if one uses a relatively blunt needle and is deliberate about the dural puncture.

The epidural space totally surrounds the dural sac and its contents and contains fatty tissue and thin-walled blood vessels. Anteriorly there are some fibrous connections between the dura and the posterior longitudinal ligament of the vertebrae. Fibrous connections are not found on the lateral and posterior surfaces, although in some cases septa, which follow fine nerve fibers to the dorsal laminae, have been noted. These septa may interfere with the distribution of local anesthetic in the epidural space.

The actual space between the ligamentum flavum and the dura varies inversely with the content of the spinal canal. The epidural space is narrow in areas with a high density of neural tissue, such as the spinal cord protuberance in the upper thoracic–lower cervical region and the bulge in the lower thoracic–upper lumbar end of the cord (both are origins of nerves going to the extremities). Once the spinal cord ends, at L2, the epidural space widens. From L2 downward, distances of from 5 to 7 mm exist between the ligamentum flavum and the dura itself. In the midthoracic region measurements of from 3 to 5 mm have been made, while in the lower cervical region the distance may be 2 mm or less. Generally, though, if the neck is flexed and the patient is in the sitting position the distance at C7, normal insertion site for a cervical spinal or epidural needle, is approximately 4 mm.

The epidural fat content is proportional to the fat in the rest of the body. Although epidural fat is for the most part free-floating, there are connected tissue septa in the more organized fat lobules. In children the fat is relatively unorganized, while in adults it is more dense. This may explain why epidural catheters are more easily advanced in children.

In addition to the spinal cord and nerves there are fine trabeculations between the pia and the arachnoid throughout the extent of the cord, creating additional barriers for the dispersion of drugs. The dentate ligaments extend laterally on either side of the cord from the pia to the arachnoid, adding stability to the position of the cord within the subarachnoid space.

The subarachnoid space exists between the arachnoid and the pia. Superiorly, the spinal subarachnoid space is connected to the cerebral subarachnoid space. Out of a total of 150 cc of cerebrospinal fluid, only 25 to 35 cc bathe the cord and cauda equina. Of this volume, about two-thirds surrounds the cervicothoracic cord while the remaining third is in the lumbar area.

The cerebrospinal fluid is an ultrafiltrate of the plasma, with which it is in equilibrium. At body temperature it has a specific gravity ranging from 1.003 to 1.009, with the average being 1.007. It exists at close to physiologic pH. CSF is formed by the choroid plexus of the lateral, third, and fourth ventricles, the majority in the lateral ventricles. The fluid thus formed bathes the spinal cord by leaving the skull via two laterally positioned foramena of Luschka and the medial foramen of Magendie. CSF returns to the bloodstream through the subarachnoid villi that project into several of the intracranial venous sinuses. A small amount of cerebrospinal fluid passes out with the spinal and cranial nerves and enters the bloodstream via capillaries and lymphatics in these structures.

Lumbar Subarachnoid Nerve Block

MIDLINE APPROACH

Single-Injection Technique

The patient is positioned on his or her side. If there is to be unilateral surgery, for example a left inguinal hernia, the side to be operated on should be down. Knees are drawn up toward the belly as much as possible. The patient's down shoulder and head are flexed toward the knees. The head is supported on a pillow. The L2 to L4 interspaces are identified by using a line between the iliac crest. This line will bisect the L4 vertebrae. The spinal tap should be attempted in the L2–L3 or L3–L4 interspaces. A 3-inch, 22- or 25-gauge spinal needle is used. Almost all spinal taps can be accomplished using a 25-gauge needle, with or without introducer. The thumb of the left hand (if the left side is down) is placed on the inferior edge of the dorsal spine above the interspace to be entered. The spinal needle is introduced through a skin wheal just below the thumb and directed slightly cephalad at a 10 to 30 degree angle. As the needle is advanced the superficial portions of the interspinous ligaments can be identified by noting increased resistance once the needle has passed through the subcutaneous tissue. The deeper layers of the interspinous ligaments and ligamentum flavum will be noted as an increased resistance when the needle is advanced in the midline. The needle then enters the epidural space, which will be felt as a sud-

den loss of resistance. The stylet is removed at this point to ascertain that there is no CSF. The stylet is then replaced and the dura arachnoid is slowly pierced. Free-flowing clear CSF will be noted in the hub of the needle.

The dose of tetracaine used may range from 6 to 15 mg (or appropriate doses of other spinal agents). Dosage depends on the site of surgery and the physical condition, hydration, age, and height of the patient. Hypo-, hyper-, or isobaric mixtures with or without a vasopressor are used for specific indications. After injection of the spinal agent, the needle is withdrawn and the patient is either maintained on his or her side for 2 to 3 minutes if the operation is to be unilateral or turned on the back if the procedure will involve both sides of the body.

If the operation involves the leg or inguinal area the spinal block is done with the patient in a 10 degree reverse Trendelenburg position. The patient is maintained in that position during the 2 to 3 minutes following needle withdrawal, assuming there is no change in sensorium or vital signs. The patient is then returned to supine position and the required anesthetic level is obtained by appropriate tilting of the table.

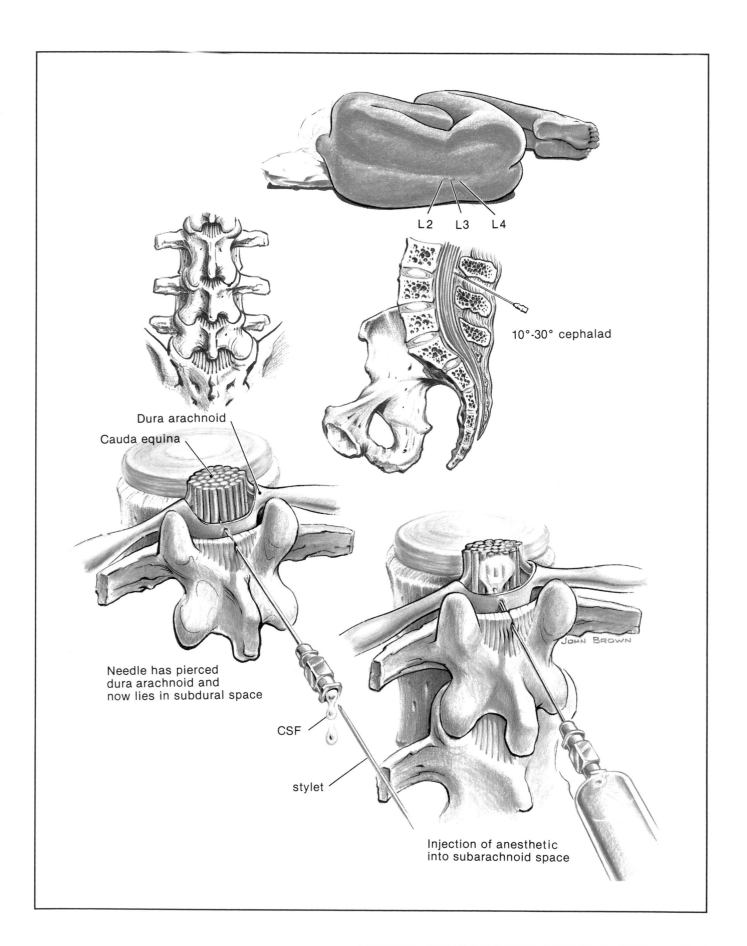

L2 L3 L4

10°-30° cephalad

Dura arachnoid

Cauda equina

Needle has pierced
dura arachnoid and
now lies in subdural space

CSF

stylet

Injection of anesthetic
into subarachnoid space

JOHN BROWN

Lumbar Subarachnoid Nerve Block

MIDLINE APPROACH

Continuous Technique

The position of the patient and identification of the correct interspace is as noted on page 170. The ligamentous structures are identified as a 17-gauge Tuohy (or similar) needle is advanced into the epidural space. The needle then pierces the dura arachnoid and enters the subarachnoid space. The stylet is partially unseated to assure that CSF flows freely. The bevel of the needle is pointed cephalad and a catheter is advanced ½ to 1 inch into the subarachnoid space. The needle is re-moved and the catheter secured in place. After the patient is returned to supine position the spinal anesthetic agent is titrated to achieve the desired anesthetic level.

Note: The catheter should not be advanced in the event of significant paresthesias. Sterile technique must be maintained at all times during the original procedure and for additional injections via the catheter.

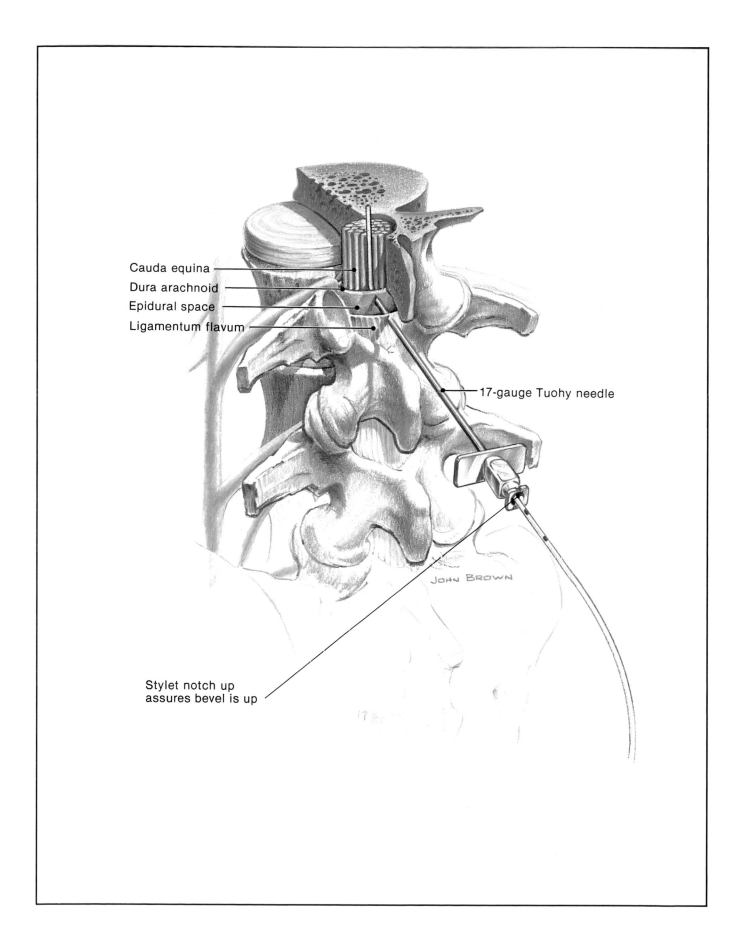

Cauda equina

Dura arachnoid

Epidural space

Ligamentum flavum

17-gauge Tuohy needle

JOHN BROWN

Stylet notch up
assures bevel is up

Lumbar Subarachnoid Nerve Block

PARAMEDIAN APPROACH

Technique

Positioning of the patient and identification of the interspaces is as noted on page 170. About 1 inch below the midline and opposite the dorsal spine of the vertebra just caudad to the interspace to be entered is the site of insertion of either a 22- or 25-gauge spinal needle. The needle is advanced so that its tip will enter the ligamentum flavum near the midline. This usually requires the needle to be inserted in a cephalad direction at approximately 30 to 45 degrees and slightly toward the medial axis of the body. Once the ligamentum flavum is identified the procedure continues as noted for the midline approach.

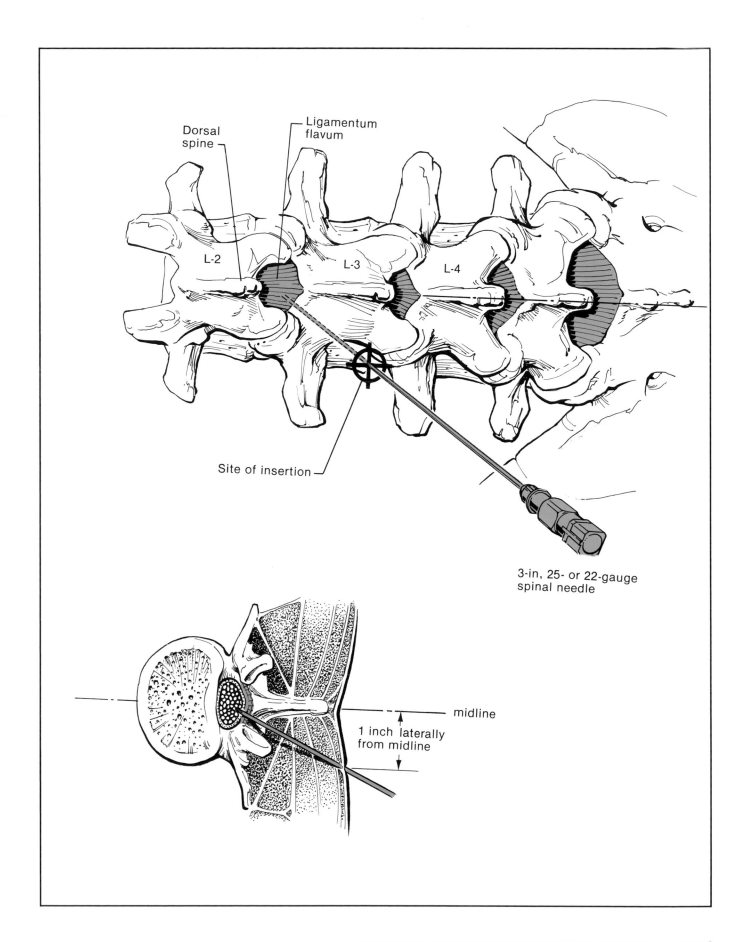

Dorsal spine

Ligamentum flavum

L-2

L-3

L-4

Site of insertion

3-in, 25- or 22-gauge spinal needle

midline

1 inch laterally from midline

Spinal Anesthetic

SADDLE BLOCK

Technique

The patient is placed in the sitting position, hands resting on knees and shoulders bent forward. A 3-inch, 25-gauge spinal needle with or without introducer is inserted through the L4–L5 interspace (see technique for spinal anesthesia on page 170). After ascertaining that the needle is in the subarachnoid space, 2 to 3 mg of tetracaine (or appropriate dose of another spinal agent) diluted with 0.5 to 1.0 cc glucose and water is injected. The patient is maintained in the sitting position for 3 to 5 minutes. In older patients this period may be extended to 7 or 8 minutes.

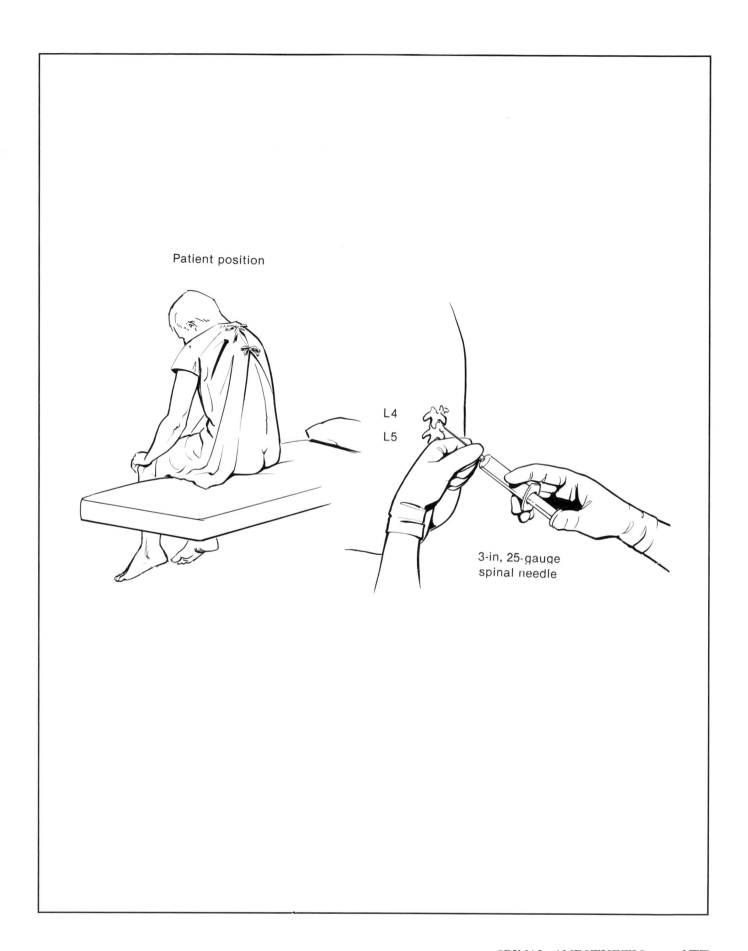

Patient position

L4
L5

3-in, 25-gauge
spinal needle

Lumbar Epidural Nerve Block

MIDLINE APPROACH

Single-Injection Technique

The patient is positioned as for a lumbar subarachnoid block (p. 170). The L3–L4 interspace is identified and the thumb of the left hand (if patient is lying left side down) is placed on the caudad portion of L3 spine. A skin wheal is raised immediately below the thumb and local anesthetic is infiltrated to a depth of about 1 inch. A 18- to 20-gauge epidural needle is advanced in a 10- to 30-degree cephalad direction using the thumb placed on the caudad portion of the dorsal spine as a guide to midline. The needle is advanced through the supraspinous ligament and into the middle layers of the interspinous ligament. At this point the stylet is removed and an air-filled glass syringe attached. The needle is then advanced through the deeper layers of the interspinous ligament and the ligamentum flavum. Continued ballottement of the syringe plunger will pro-duce increasing resistance as the deeper layers of the ligaments are entered. When the needle tip pierces the ligamentum flavum there will be a sudden loss of resistance. Four cubic centimeters of local anesthetic with epinephrine 1:200,000 is then injected. After ensuring that neither intravascular nor intrathecal injection has occurred, the definitive dose of local anesthetic, usually 1 to 2 cc per dermatome to be blocked, is injected. The needle is removed and, assuming bilateral anesthesia is required, the patient is returned to the supine position.

Note: If unilateral anesthesia is desired the patient should be positioned with the side to be blocked down and remain in that position for several minutes after the definitive dose of local anesthetic is injected.

Continuous Technique

The patient is positioned as for a spinal anesthetic (p. 170) and the procedure is performed exactly like a lumbar epidural midline single-injection block except that a 17- or 18-gauge, thin-wall epidural needle is used. After the epidural space has been entered an appropriate catheter is advanced ½ to 1 inch past the tip of the needle. The needle is removed and the catheter secured in place. A 4 cc test dose of local anesthetic with epinephrine 1:200,000 is injected. After ensuring that the catheter tip is neither intravascular nor intrathecal the definitive dose of 1 to 2 cc per dermatome to be blocked is injected.

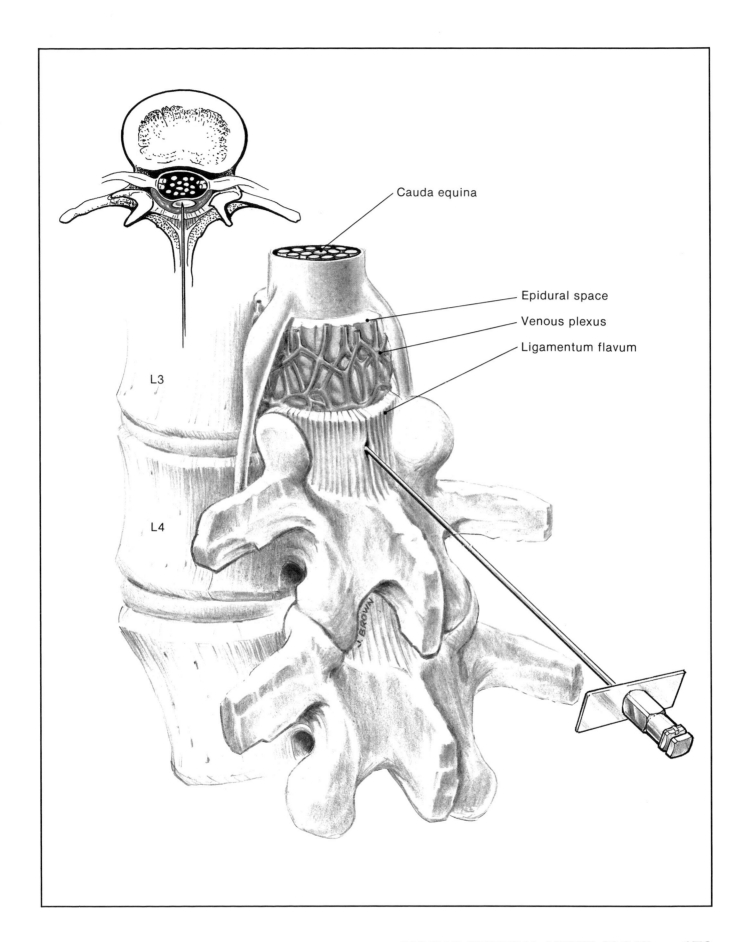

Cauda equina

Epidural space

Venous plexus

Ligamentum flavum

L3

L4

J. BROWN

Lumbar Epidural Nerve Block

PARAMEDIAN APPROACH

Technique

The patient is positioned as for a lumbar subarachnoid nerve block (p. 170) and the L3–L4 interspace is identified. A skin wheal is made 1 to 1½ inches lateral to the midline at a point parallel to the caudal aspect of the dorsal spine of the L3 vertebrae. An epidural needle, either 18- to 20-gauge for single-shot or 17- to 18-gauge thin-wall for continuous injections, is inserted at an angle of approximately 10 degrees toward the midline and 30 to 45 degrees cephalad. The needle is advanced into the soft tissue and an air-filled glass syringe attached. Gentle ballottement will note minimal resistance as the needle advances through the soft paraspinous tissues until it reaches the ligamentum flavum. At this point the resistance to ballottement will markedly increase. The needle tip will then pierce the ligamentum flavum and enter the epidural space. The procedure continues as described for the lumbar epidural midline approach single-injection or continuous block (p. 178).

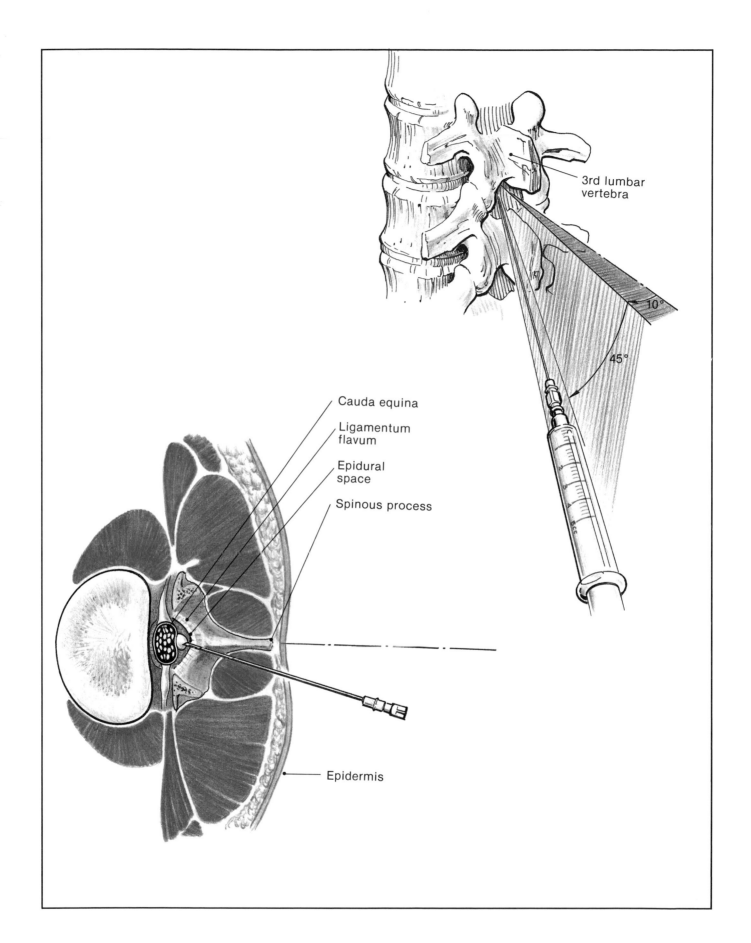

3rd lumbar
vertebra

10°

45°

Cauda equina

Ligamentum
flavum

Epidural
space

Spinous process

Epidermis

Thoracic Subarachnoid Nerve Block

MIDLINE APPROACH

Technique

The patient lies in the lateral position with the head comfortably resting on a pillow. The thorax is bowed out toward the operator. For midthoracic spinal blocks the angulation of the dorsal spines is very acute and the interspaces are relatively narrow. The appropriate dorsal spine is identified by counting down from the cervical area or up from the lumbar area. A 3- to 3½-inch, 22-gauge spinal needle is inserted at an acute angle in the interspinous space. The operator should have the feel of the ligamentous structures being penetrated by the needle when it is in the midline. As deeper layers of the ligaments are met, resistance to the advancing needle will increase slightly. Two endpoints should be encountered when a 22-gauge needle is used: (1) the entrance of the needle into the epidural space, which will be noted as a slight loss of resistance, and (2) the puncture of the dura arachnoid. The first endpoint should be identified by removing the stylet from the needle and ascertaining that no CSF can be withdrawn. The second endpoint, which is usually obvious, should produce a free flow of CSF.

For blocks done below the level of T9 the acuteness of the angle of needle insertion is modified and the technique is essentially the same as described for blocks in the lumbar area.

For correct doses of local anesthetics see cervical subarachnoid nerve block (p. 192).

Note: Since there is so little space between the dura arachnoid and the substance of the spinal cord, they should be punctured by advancing the needle very slowly.

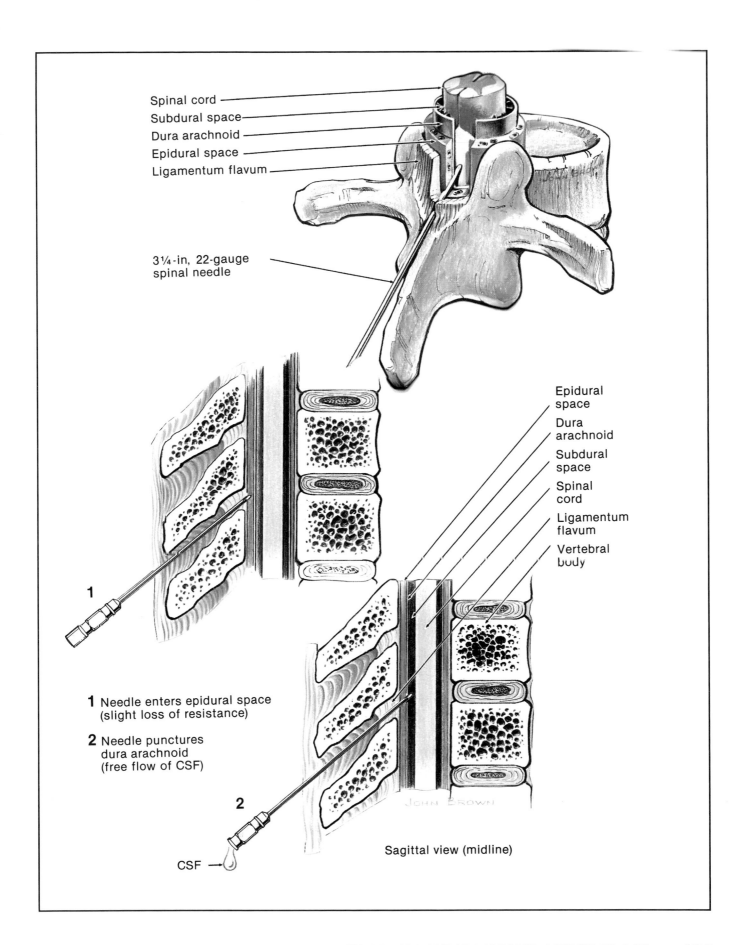

Spinal cord

Subdural space

Dura arachnoid

Epidural space

Ligamentum flavum

3¼-in, 22-gauge
spinal needle

Epidural
space

Dura
arachnoid

Subdural
space

Spinal
cord

Ligamentum
flavum

Vertebral
body

1 Needle enters epidural space
(slight loss of resistance)

2 Needle punctures
dura arachnoid
(free flow of CSF)

CSF →

Sagittal view (midline)

JOHN BROWN

Thoracic Subarachnoid Nerve Block

PARAMEDIAN APPROACH

Technique

Position of the patient and location of the appropriate interspace is the same as noted for thoracic subarachnoid—midline approach (p. 182). At a point approximately ½ to 1 inch lateral to the inferior edge of the dorsal spine of the interspace to be entered, a 3½-inch, 22-gauge spinal needle is inserted, pointing cephalad at a 45- to 50-degree angle. The needle is also directed toward the midline in hope of piercing the dura at the center of the interspace.

The lamina of a thoracic vertebra may be encountered before the interspace is entered, in which case the needle is directed slightly more cephalad and medially. Once deep to the lamina the needle should be advanced slowly until the dura arachnoid is punctured and CSF appears at the needle hub.

The puncture of the dura arachnoid is usually an obvious and distinct endpoint. The dosage regimen to be used for both diagnostic and therapeutic purposes is similar to that described for cervical subarachnoid nerve block (p. 192.)

Note: Since the spinal cord lies immediately under it, piercing the dura arachnoid should be done very deliberately. To ascertain that the hub of the needle is entirely within the CSF, *gentle* aspiration is done, which should produce a free flow of fluid.

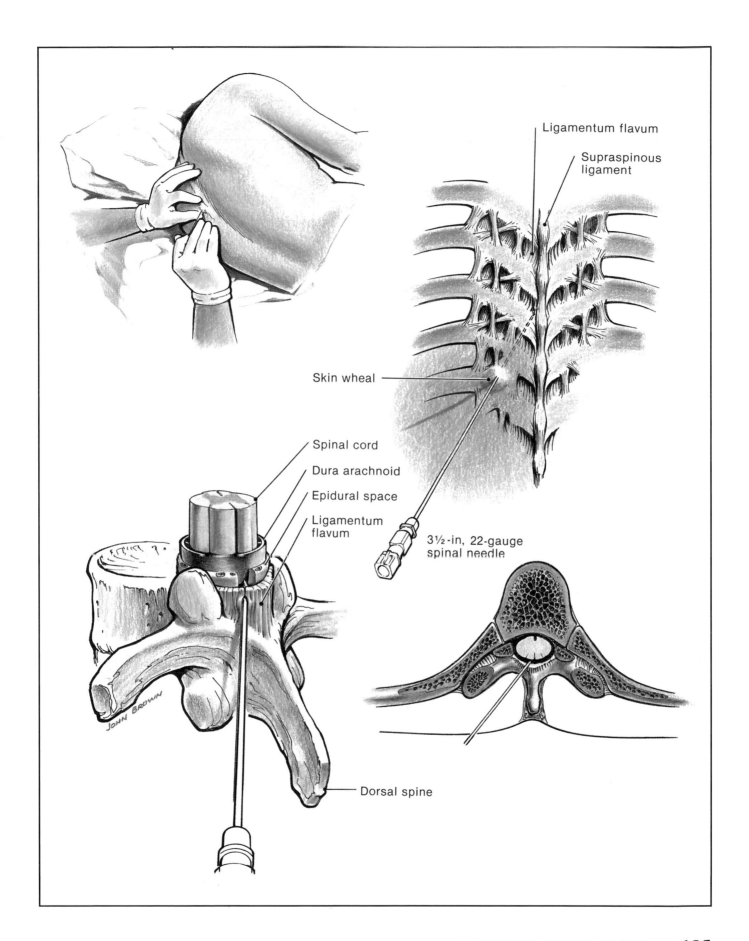

Ligamentum flavum

Supraspinous
ligament

Skin wheal

Spinal cord

Dura arachnoid

Epidural space

Ligamentum
flavum

3½-in, 22-gauge
spinal needle

JOHN BROWN

Dorsal spine

Thoracic Epidural Nerve Block

MIDLINE APPROACH

Single-Injection Technique

Since the positioning and technique resemble a thoracic subarachnoid block, see also pages 182 and 184. For single-injection thoracic epidural blocks an 18- to 20-gauge, thin-wall needle is inserted in the midline at a very acute angle of from 35 to 60 degrees. The loss-of-resistance technique is used to identify the epidural space. The interspinous ligaments and ligamentum flavum can be identified by noting the increased resistance to ballottement of the plunger of an air-filled glass syringe as the needle is advanced through the interspace. There is a sudden loss of resistance when the epidural space is entered. A test dose of 2 to 3 cc of local anesthetic with epinephrine 1:200,000 to rule out intrathecal or intravascular injection is given. Usually 1 cc or less of local anesthetic per thoracic dermatome to be blocked is then injected and the patient is turned supine immediately.

Note: See the precautions on page 188.

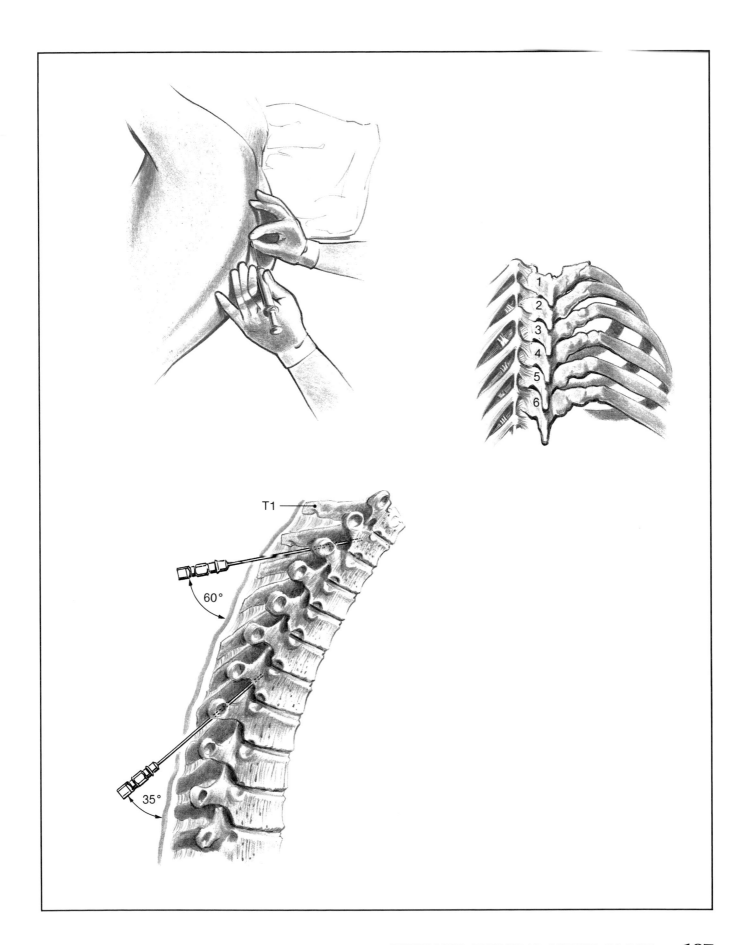

Thoracic Epidural Nerve Block

MIDLINE APPROACH

Continuous Technique

The technique is as for thoracic epidural—midline approach single-injection, with some exceptions. A 17-gauge, thin-wall Tuohy or similar needle is used. After identification of the epidural space the bevel of the needle is directed cephalad. A catheter is then advanced ½ to 1 inch beyond the end of the needle. The needle is removed and the catheter secured in place. A test dose of 2 to 3 cc of local anesthetic with epinephrine 1:200,000 is injected to rule out intravascular or intrathecal injection. The definitive dose of local anesthetic will be 1 cc or less per thoracic dermatome to be blocked.

Note: Since the space between the spines is very narrow and their angulation quite severe, the midline approach may be difficult. As the spinal cord is immediately under the dura arachnoid, this technique must be done deliberately, with absolute identification of the ligaments.

Note: For blocks done below T9 the technique is much simpler, in essence the same as that described for lumbar epidural block on page 178.

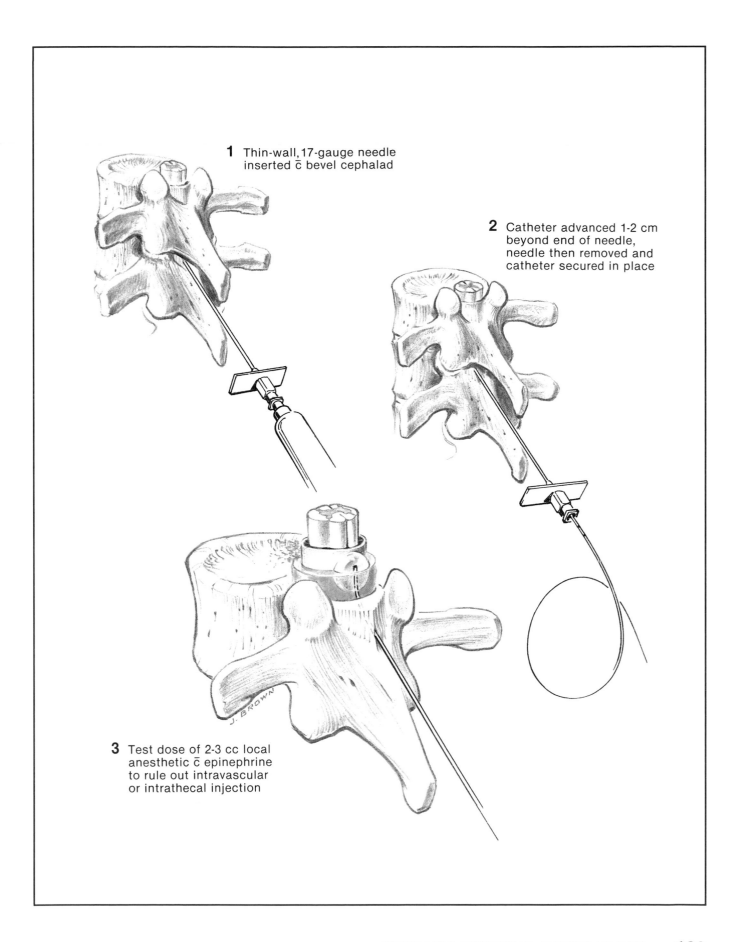

1 Thin-wall,17-gauge needle inserted c̄ bevel cephalad

2 Catheter advanced 1-2 cm beyond end of needle, needle then removed and catheter secured in place

3 Test dose of 2-3 cc local anesthetic c̄ epinephrine to rule out intravascular or intrathecal injection

Thoracic Epidural Nerve Block

PARAMEDIAN APPROACH

Technique

The patient is positioned as for the thoracic subarachnoid nerve block (p. 182). The dorsal spine of the appropriate interspace is identified by counting down from C7 or up from the lumbar area. One-half to one inch lateral to the caudad border of the spine a skin wheal is raised. After adequate infiltration with local anesthetic, a 3½-inch, 18- to 20-gauge epidural needle is inserted perpendicular to the skin. The vertebral arch of the immediate caudad vertebra is contacted. The needle is then redirected cephalad and slightly medially until bone contact is lost. The tip of the needle should then be immediately above the ligamentum flavum. A glass syringe filled with air is attached and the needle is advanced into the ligament. Ballottement of the plunger will show increased resistance as the hub of the needle enters the substance of the ligament. The needle is then slowly advanced, with continuous ballottement of the plunger, until a sudden loss of resistance occurs, indicating that the tip of the needle has pierced the ligament and now lies in the epidural space.

After careful aspiration a 3-cc test dose of local anesthetic with epinephrine 1:200,000 is injected. After ensuring that the test dose is neither subarachnoid nor intravascular, the definitive dose of local anesthetic, 1 cc or less per dermatome, is injected slowly. The patient is returned to the supine position immediately after the needle is removed.

If a catheter technique is to be used, after the epidural space has been identified the needle bevel is directed cephalad. An appropriate catheter is then advanced ½ to 1 inch beyond the bevel and secured in place. A test dose of 3 cc of local anesthetic with epinephrine 1:200,000 is injected after careful aspiration. After ensuring that the catheter is neither intravascular nor in the subarachnoid space, the definitive dose, also 1 cc or less per dermatome, is injected.

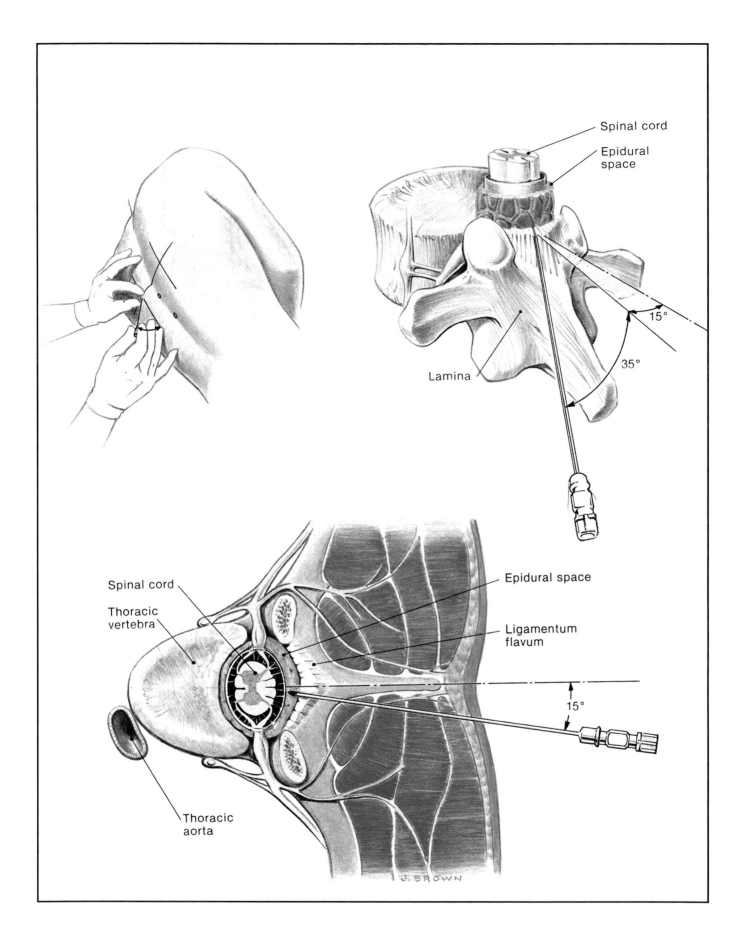

Spinal cord

Epidural space

15°

35°

Lamina

Spinal cord

Thoracic vertebra

Epidural space

Ligamentum flavum

15°

Thoracic aorta

J. BROWN

THORACIC EPIDURAL NERVE BLOCK   **191**

Cervical Subarachnoid Nerve Block

Technique

The patient lies in the lateral position with the head supported on a pillow so that the axis of the spinal cord remains straight. The head is flexed forward. The C6 or C7 interspace is chosen and a 3-inch, 22-gauge spinal needle is advanced perpendicular to the axis of the vertebral column in the midline. The needle passes through the well-developed nuchal ligaments and into the easily identified epidural space. The stylet of the spinal needle is withdrawn to confirm that the tip of the needle is in the epidural space (as evidenced by absence of CSF in the needle), then replaced. The needle is slowly advanced until the dura arachnoid is pierced.

For diagnostic purposes, 1 mg of tetracaine (or similar dose of another spinal anesthetic) in 1 cc of sterile water is injected; for therapeutic procedures (i.e., surgery), 2 to 5 mg of tetracaine (or similar dose of another spinal anesthetic) in a hyperbaric solution with dextrose in water will provide anesthesia for the neck, arm, and upper thorax.

Note: The needle should be advanced very slowly through the epidural space and into the subarachnoid space. CSF will appear in the needle tip and should flow freely with *gentle* aspiration prior to injection.

Note: Systemic hypotension should be anticipated and appropriate therapy instituted as required. Although unlikely, it is possible that respiratory depression or apnea will occur with this technique. Appropriate means for respiratory assistance and oxygenation must be available.

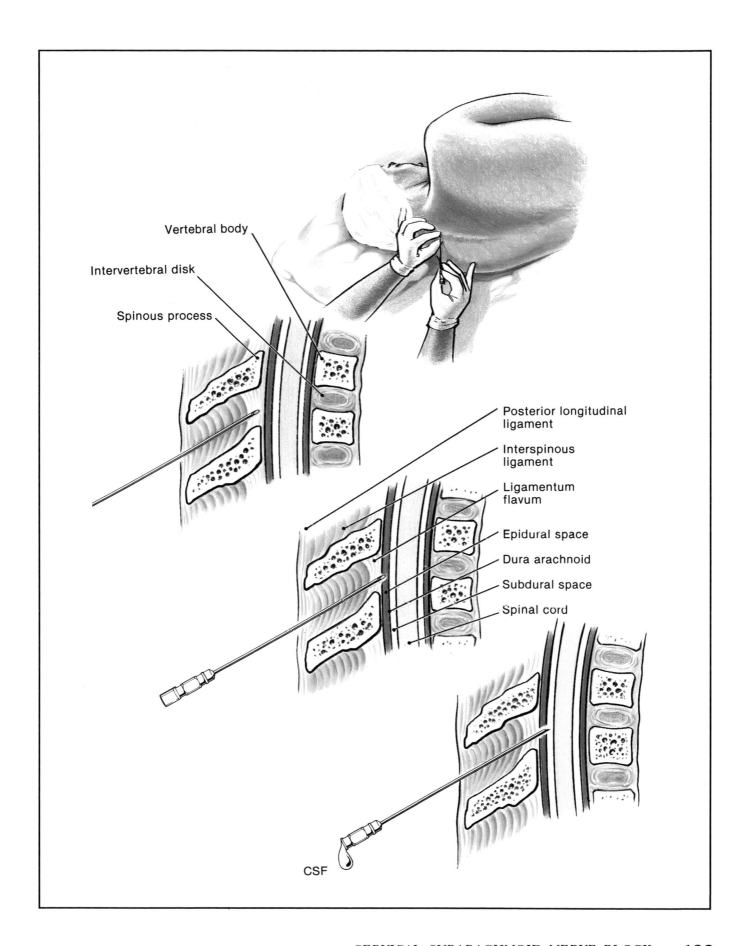

Vertebral body

Intervertebral disk

Spinous process

Posterior longitudinal ligament

Interspinous ligament

Ligamentum flavum

Epidural space

Dura arachnoid

Subdural space

Spinal cord

CSF

Cervical Epidural Nerve Block

Single Injection Technique

This block is done with the patient sitting, head flexed forward, and is best accomplished using the "hanging-drop" technique. For a single-injection cervical epidural block, an 18- to 20-gauge epidural needle is inserted in the midline at the C6 or C7 interspace perpendicular to the spine. With the stylet in place the needle is slowly advanced into the ligaments. The stylet is then removed and the needle hub filled with sterile saline so that a hanging drop is evident. The needle is then slowly advanced into the epidural space, which is identified when the fluid is sucked in.

This end point, with the patient in the sitting position, is very dramatic and quite obvious to the operator. After careful and gentle aspiration a dose of local anesthetic sufficient to cover the required dermatomes is injected. This dose will vary from 1 to 2 cc per dermatome (occasionally less), depending on the physical condition and age of the patient.

Continuous Technique

The positioning is as above. A 17-gauge, thin-wall Tuohy or similar needle is advanced into the epidural space using the hanging-drop technique. The bevel of the needle should be pointed in a cephalad direction prior to advancing the catheter ½ to 1 inch beyond the tip of the needle. The catheter is then secured in the usual manner. A test dose of 2 to 3 cc of local anesthetic with epinephrine 1:200,000 is injected after the patient is returned to the supine position. In the absence of signs of systemic vascular absorption or inadvertent intrathecal injection, the definitive dose of local anesthetic, 1 to 2 cc per dermatone or occasionally less, depending on the physical condition and age of the patient, is injected. Timing of repeat injections depends on the local anesthetic used. In general, injections will be required every 45 to 90 minutes in amounts approximately 50 percent that of the initial injection.

Note: Systemic hypotension should be anticipated and appropriate therapy instituted as required. Although unlikely, it is possible that respiratory depression or apnea will occur with this technique. Appropriate means for respiratory assistance and oxygenation must be available.

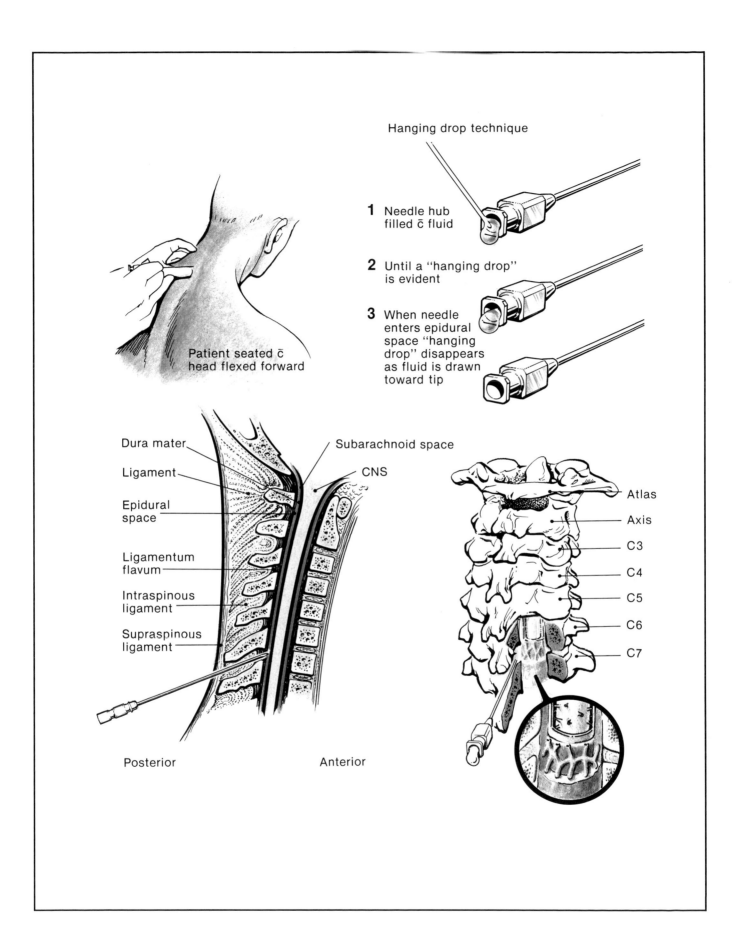

Hanging drop technique

1 Needle hub filled c̄ fluid

2 Until a "hanging drop" is evident

3 When needle enters epidural space "hanging drop" disappears as fluid is drawn toward tip

Patient seated c̄ head flexed forward

Dura mater

Ligament

Epidural space

Ligamentum flavum

Intraspinous ligament

Supraspinous ligament

Subarachnoid space

CNS

Posterior

Anterior

Atlas

Axis

C3

C4

C5

C6

C7

Index

Page numbers in italics indicate an illustration.

Ventral roots, 100
Vertebrae, 100
  typical, 168
Vertebral artery and convulsions, 50
Vertebral column, 94, 108, 168
Vocal cords, 52, 56; *see also* Larynx

Wrist, 76
  median nerve block at, 86–87
  radial nerve block at, 84–85
  ulnar nerve block at, 88–89

X-ray/radiologic verification of needle-tip placement, 4,
  94, 96, 108, 110, 112

Zygomatic arch, 12, *13*, 18, *19*
Zygomaticofacial branch of maxillary division, 2
Zygomaticotemporal branch of maxillary division, 2